"Lisa Shetler understands the whirlwind of emotions and c
the perfect guide to help them navigate it all. Full of enga
Mental Health in Middle School gives kids a safe space to learn how to navigate friendships and
manage their thoughts and feelings. Fun, insightful, and empowering, this workbook is a must-have
tool for any middle schooler looking to build their resilience in these crucial years!"

—**Phyllis L. Fagell**, licensed therapist, school counselor, and author of **Middle School Matters** and
Middle School Superpowers

"Lisa Shetler provides a wealth of tools to help preteens navigate the challenges of these years in a way
that is fun and engaging—replete with drawings, games, and comics. What is particularly unique and
refreshing in this book is the consistent inclusion of written-out, 'how-to' messages that preteens could
take directly to the adults in their lives, rather than struggle to find the right words to ask for help. So
needed! This is an absolute must-have book for any preteens in your life!"

—**Karen Bluth, PhD,** professor emerita at University of North Carolina; and author of **The
Self-Compassionate Workbook for Teens**, **The Self-Compassionate Teen**, and **Mindful Self-
Compassion for Teens in Schools**

"An informative, practical, easy-to-read guide on how to survive and thrive in middle school. Every kid
would benefit from learning these skills and strategies—as would their parents. If you want to help your
child face their fears, tackle their challenges, overcome their obstacles, build friendships, grow as a
person, and generally get the most out of life—give them this book. You won't regret it."

—**Russ Harris**, author of **The Happiness Trap** and **ACT Made Simple**

"Lisa's expertise and creative approach to helping children build essential life skills is well demonstrated
in her workbook. This beautifully crafted series of exercises promises to help young people develop
insight and build tools that are fundamental to their self-care. These very tools can support children in
learning from their mistakes, build resilience in a rapidly changing world, and connect more deeply to
themselves. This workbook is a must for all preteens."

—**Lorraine M. Hobbs, MA,** founding director of youth and family programs at University of
California, San Diego's Center for Mindfulness; and author of **Teaching Self-Compassion to
Teens** and **The Self-Compassion Workbook for Kids**

"*Mastering Your Mental Health in Middle School* is a wonderful workbook, packed full of important skills which are designed to empower preteens, help them navigate challenges, and cope with a wide range of feelings. If you are a parent/caregiver of a preteen, or a therapist working with preteens, I highly recommend this workbook for preteens."

—**Tamar D. Black, PhD,** educational and developmental psychologist, and author of *ACT for Treating Children* and *The ACT Workbook for Kids*

"Lisa Shetler has written with warmth and wisdom, offering a nurturing space where young readers can slow down, reflect, and explore their inner world with compassion and curiosity. Her thoughtful guidance gently invites discovery, awareness, and self-acceptance, which can sometimes feel elusive during a time of such change and growth."

—**Karen Young, (MGestTher),** neurodevelopment consultant, director of Hey Sigmund, and author of *Hey Warrior*

"Read the book and learn to climb the Mount Everest that is adolescence! That's what is in this fun book for teens. Easy to read, fun images, language that is engaging, and exercises that can be used alone or with the support of adults. Parents and professionals will find this a fabulous resource to share."

—**Louise Hayes,** developer of the DNA-V model of acceptance and commitment therapy (ACT) for youth, and author of *Your Life Your Way* and *What Makes You Stronger*

MASTERING *Your* MENTAL HEALTH *in* MIDDLE SCHOOL

A Workbook to Deal with Stress, Manage Intense Emotions, Boost Confidence & Cope with Whatever Comes Your Way

LISA SHETLER, MPSYCH

Instant Help Books
An Imprint of New Harbinger Publications, Inc.

Publisher's Note

This publication is designed to provide accurate and authoritative information in regard to the subject matter covered. It is sold with the understanding that the publisher is not engaged in rendering psychological, financial, legal, or other professional services. If expert assistance or counseling is needed, the services of a competent professional should be sought.

INSTANT HELP, the Clock Logo, and NEW HARBINGER are trademarks of New Harbinger Publications, Inc.

New Harbinger Publications is an employee-owned company.

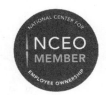

Copyright © 2025 by Lisa Shetler

Instant Help Books

An imprint of New Harbinger Publications, Inc.

5720 Shattuck Avenue

Oakland, CA 94609

www.newharbinger.com

Cover design by Amy Shoup

Interior design by Tom Comitta

Acquired by Tesilya Hanauer

Edited by Callie Brown

Printed in the United States of America

27   26   25

10   9   8   7   6   5   4   3   2   1   First Printing

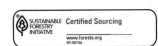

CONTENTS

ACKNOWLEDGMENTS

I acknowledge the Kaurna people as the Traditional Owners and Custodians of the land on which I reside and work, and on which I wrote this book. May the strength of your people, the wisdom of your culture, and the beauty of your land continue to provide healing from the past and a path forward to a bright future for all young people.

To the team at New Harbinger Publications, particularly Tesilya Hanauer and Callie Brown: Thank you for seeing the need for resources tailored to preteens and for supporting this project with such wisdom and warmth.

To the team at Flow Psychology and Therapeutic Services, who work skillfully and passionately with young people and families every day: You constantly inspire me with your courage, creativity, and compassion. Thank you for helping this book grow out of the work you do.

To my family, chosen family, mentors, and friends: Thank you for your unending support, guidance, encouragement, belief, and patience. I would not be who I am, doing what I love to do, without each and every one of you.

To every young person who has sat in my office: Thank you for sharing your lives, stories, struggles, and strengths with me. May you all lead wonderful, meaningful, fulfilling lives.

NOTE FOR PARENTS, CAREGIVERS, AND HELPERS

I am delighted you have found your way to this workbook, which is designed to help preteens master essential skills for managing their mental health.

In today's rapidly evolving world, preteens are faced with an overwhelming array of challenges. The transition from childhood to adolescence inevitably brings about significant changes—physical, emotional, and mental. It's perhaps not surprising, then, that the number of preteens facing significant mental illness is, unfortunately, increasing.

This workbook aims to empower young people with knowledge and skills to understand and manage their emotions, build resilience, and develop both healthy relationships and a healthy mindset. It offers practical tools and insights to navigate the unique challenges of being a preteen and the complex task of growing up.

THE CHALLENGES PRETEENS FACE

Preteens (ages eight to twelve) are at a critical stage of development. They experience emotional fluctuations, new social pressures, academic demands, and questions of identity. And then there's puberty!

EMOTIONAL FLUCTUATIONS As their brains develop, preteens can experience intense and often confusing emotions. They're learning to identify and express more complex feelings and are grappling with more serious issues and demands.

SOCIAL PRESSURES The social-emotional maturity of preteens varies. Exposure to mature content may take you and them by surprise. Childhood friendships change, sometimes dramatically. Social dynamics in preteens' peer groups become more complex, and they can experience increased pressure to fit in along with more peer conflict, including bullying.

ACADEMIC DEMANDS As kids transition to middle school, academic expectations rise, leading to increased stress and anxiety about performance and future prospects. Perfectionistic tendencies can surface, and preteens may struggle with unrealistic expectations, negative comparisons, and low self-worth.

IDENTITY EXPLORATION Preteens are starting to explore their identities, which involves questioning their values, beliefs, and place in the world. They may express ideas that are different from those they have been raised with and look more to external influences to shape their beliefs.

PUBERTY! The visible physical changes are just at the surface of the immense development preteens' brains and bodies are undergoing. There may be shame, embarrassment, fear, and discomfort associated with bodily changes.

All these factors, coupled with the influence of technology and social media, mean preteens must develop robust skills to support their mental health.

HOW TO HELP A PRETEEN USE THIS WORKBOOK

This workbook provides educational content, reflective exercises, and practical activities. Here's how to help a preteen make the most of it.

ENGAGE ACTIVELY The skills in this workbook will be most effective when practiced regularly and incorporated into daily life over time. Help preteens apply the skills by talking about the exercises, modeling them, and even doing them together.

CREATE A SAFE SPACE Your support and encouragement are crucial. Encourage preteens to express their thoughts and feelings by reminding them they are great just as they are, and by being willing to listen (not fix). Show them you are interested in getting to know them—their friends, values, interests—even if you don't always agree.

TAKE THEIR EXPERIENCE SERIOUSLY Throughout the workbook are tools designed to help your preteen capture data about their wellbeing (sleep tracker, mood tracker, skill tracker, and wellbeing and health check). There's a help request card they can tear out to help them start difficult conversations—including with you. If they tell you they're struggling, please believe them, and recruit any additional support needed.

RESPECT THEIR PACE Every preteen is unique. Allow them to progress at their own pace, including pausing and revisiting sections of the workbook as needed.

Trusted adults play a vital role in guiding preteens through this phase of their development. Connection is the single greatest protective factor young people can have against mental health struggles. Your involvement, understanding, and support matter. Together, we can equip the young minds in our care with the skills they need to thrive.

Most sincerely,

Lisa Shetler

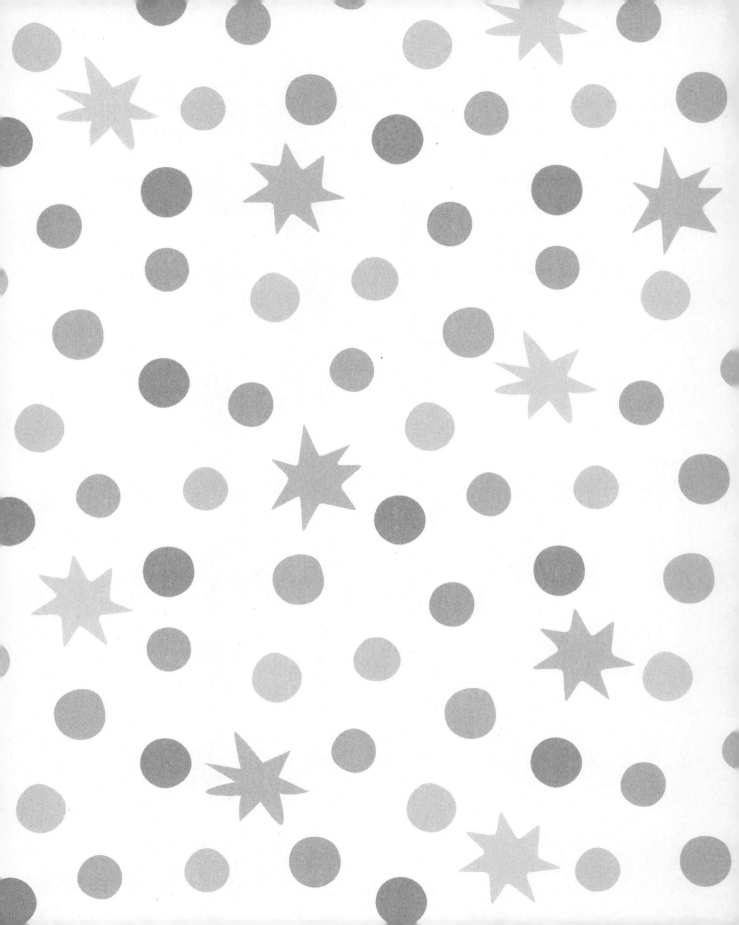

MASTERY

(noun)

Knowledge and skill that allow you to use, do, or understand something very well.

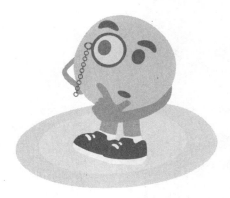

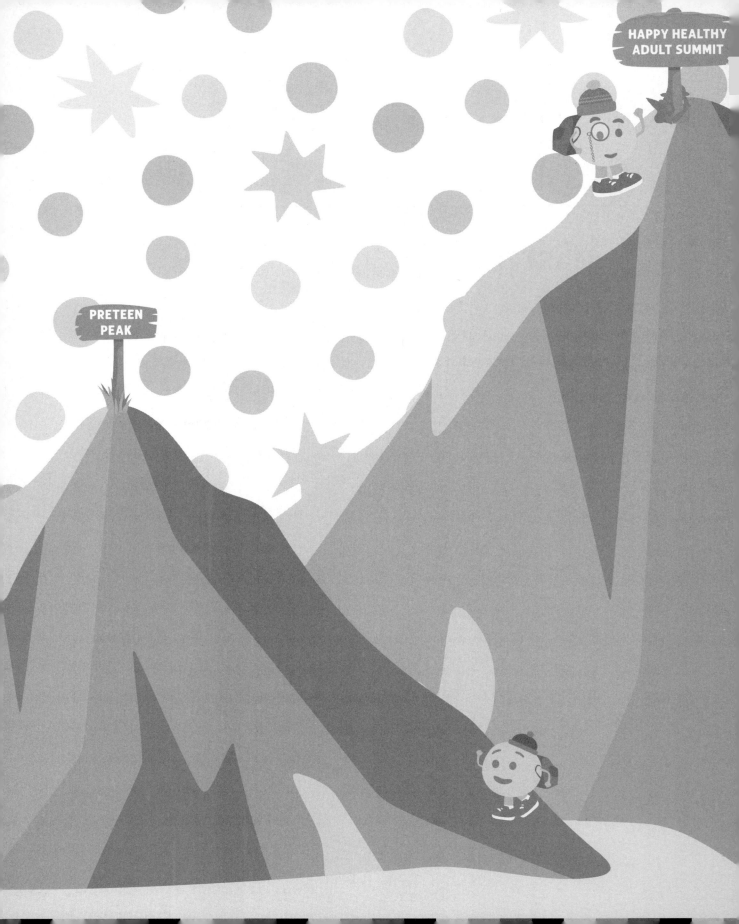

Chapter 1

WELCOME TO THE JOURNEY

I'm glad you're here! Middle school is a journey, and this book is here to help you as you travel. If you're struggling with some things at school, at home, with friends, or within yourself, someone clever (maybe you) thought this workbook could help. Good news: It can!

THE MOUNTAIN: A SYMBOL OF CHALLENGE AND STRENGTH

Imagine standing at the foot of a majestic mountain. Its peaks rise into the clouds, inviting you to climb to the very top. The mountain represents your journey toward being a teenager—a time filled with excitement, challenges, and self-discovery.

Looking at what's ahead can also feel like a lot! As you climb, you'll find rough ground, unpredictable weather, and fellow climbers on their own journey. From where you're standing, it might be hard to see how you're going to make it to the top.

Even experienced mountaineers need a guide—someone who's climbed the mountain and can help show the way. I'm an expert at helping young people just like you make it to the summit, and I wrote this workbook to be your guide.

Climbing a mountain takes skill, perseverance, and ability to manage tough days and enjoy great ones. This workbook will help you master skills like:

- taking good care of yourself and managing thoughts and feelings

- handling issues with friends

- picking yourself up when things don't go as planned

You'll climb the cliffs of self-confidence and navigate the fog of uncertainty. You'll add tools to your pack that will help you overcome any obstacle. The view from the top will be worth the effort, and the skills you learn will be yours for life.

So grab your backpack of curiosity and courage and get ready for adventure—your path to the top starts here!

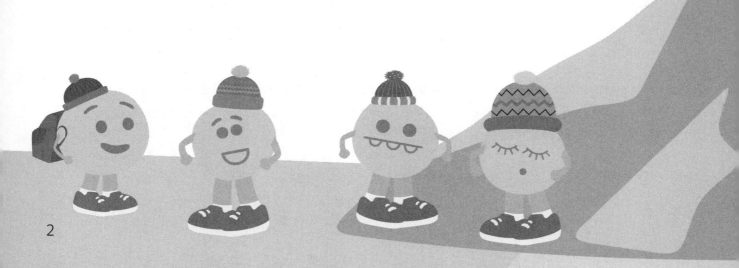

PRETEEN PEAK:
A GLIMPSE OF WHAT'S POSSIBLE

Have you heard of Mount Everest's base camp? It's where climbers prepare for what's ahead. Right now, you're at Preteen Peak—a base camp where you'll gear up for the climb into your teen years and beyond. Just like adventurers preparing to climb mountains, preteens can build skills, gear up, and study maps to plan the journey.

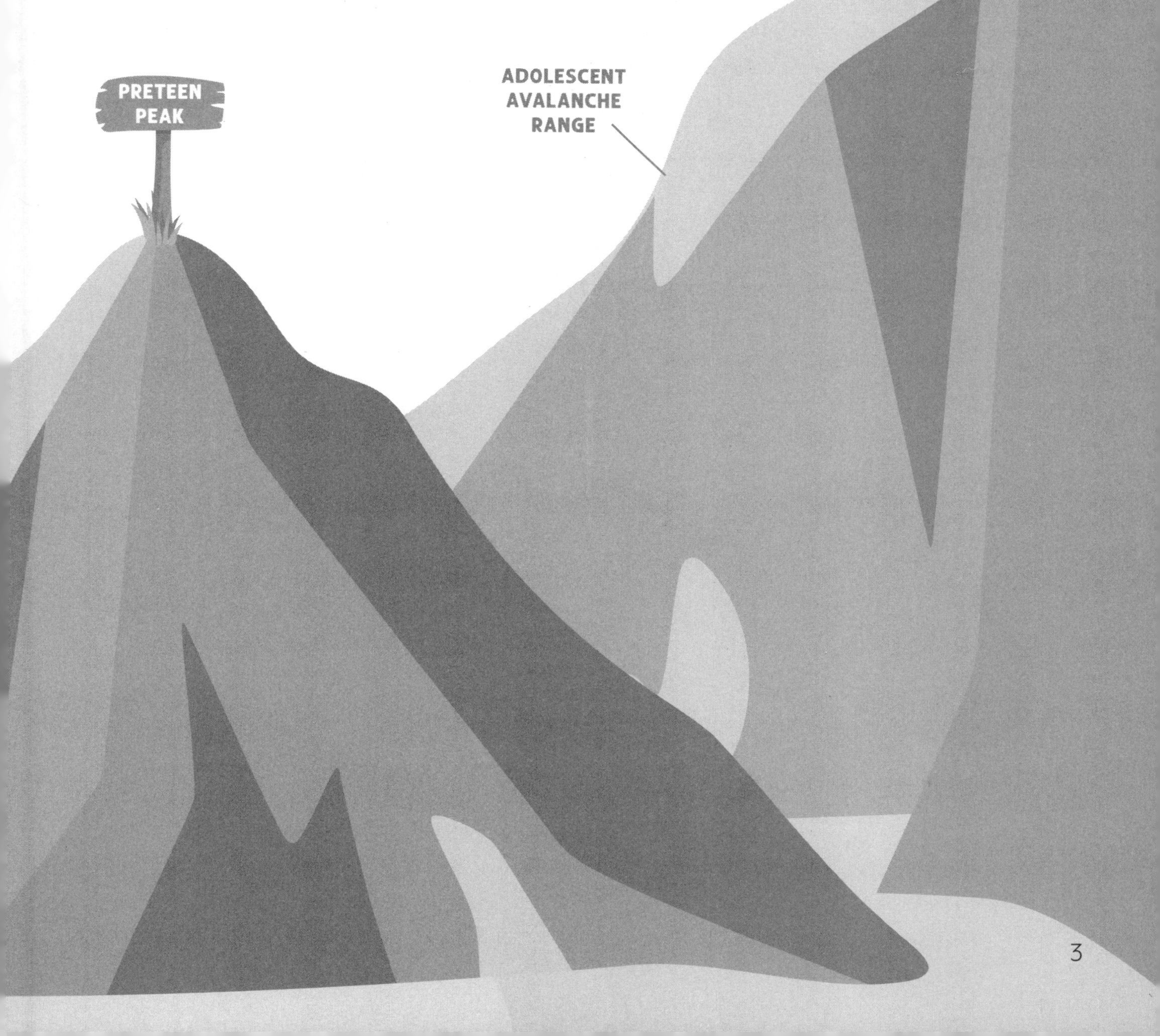

HAPPY HEALTHY ADULT SUMMIT

ADOLESCENT AVALANCHE RANGE

PRETEEN PEAK

Preteen Peak is about preparing for the "adolescent avalanche," when the terrain starts shifting and old snow tumbles away. Lots of things change—sometimes all at once! Sometimes the path will feel long or hard. Maybe you're facing struggles at school or home. Maybe things with friends are changing. Or maybe your thoughts and feelings are getting the best of you. You might wish you could turn back or give up!

But trust me: The view from the summit is worth it. You'll be up there living your best life, surrounded by people who love and accept you—and one of them is you. It may be hard to believe right now, but one day you'll look back proudly. You'll see how far you've come, and the challenges you're facing now will feel far away. Preteen Peak will help you learn skills to live your best life. Visualizing yourself at the mountaintop as an awesome young adult will inspire you to keep going, even when things get tough.

Let's start with an activity to get you thinking about your future.

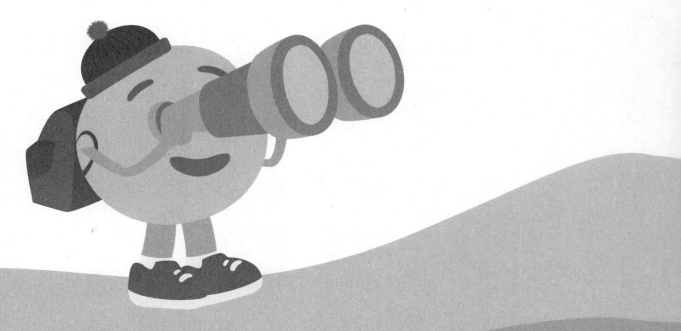

YOUR VISION BOARD

Your Vision Board is a personalized reminder of your hopes, dreams, and goals. It will encourage you on the tough days and keep you focused on moving forward.

1. **GATHERING YOUR GEAR.** Find a blank canvas for your board: a posterboard, a notebook, or a digital document.

2. **IMAGINING YOURSELF.** You're a young adult at the top of your mountain. You're a bit older and wiser, and you're filled with the joy of reaching your goals. What does success look like for you? What makes you happy? What do you feel proud to have achieved?

3. **ARTISTIC EXPEDITION.** Now get creative! Draw, cut and paste, or make a digital collage that's a vision of future you on the mountaintop. Choose words or images that show:

   - what success looks like
   - what the important things in your life are
   - what strengths you have that help you conquer challenges

4. **PEAK PERFECTION.** Display your masterpiece somewhere you'll see it every day— your bedroom wall or your screen wallpaper. As you climb, you can add to your board. It's your own gallery of hopes and dreams!

As you gear up at Preteen Peak and the adventure begins, your Vision Board will inspire you to conquer whatever challenges come.

PREPARING FOR THE JOURNEY AHEAD

As you navigate the adolescent avalanche and a fulfilling, healthy adult life, let's get clear about what skills you need!

Below, write what strengths you think a mountain climber needs. Is it courage when things are uncertain? Persistence when times are tough? A sense of humor when things go wrong? What else?

_____

_____

_____

_____

The unknown can feel scary. Below, write down any fears or worries you have about journeying through middle school and into the teenage years.

_____

_____

_____

_____

In the next chapter, we'll figure out which skills you already have—and which you can learn—to help you navigate your middle school years.

BONUS ACTIVITY Ask people close to you what they think your greatest strengths are. Write their answers here:

_____

_____

_____

_____

_____

_____

_____

_____

_____

_____

_____

_____

_____

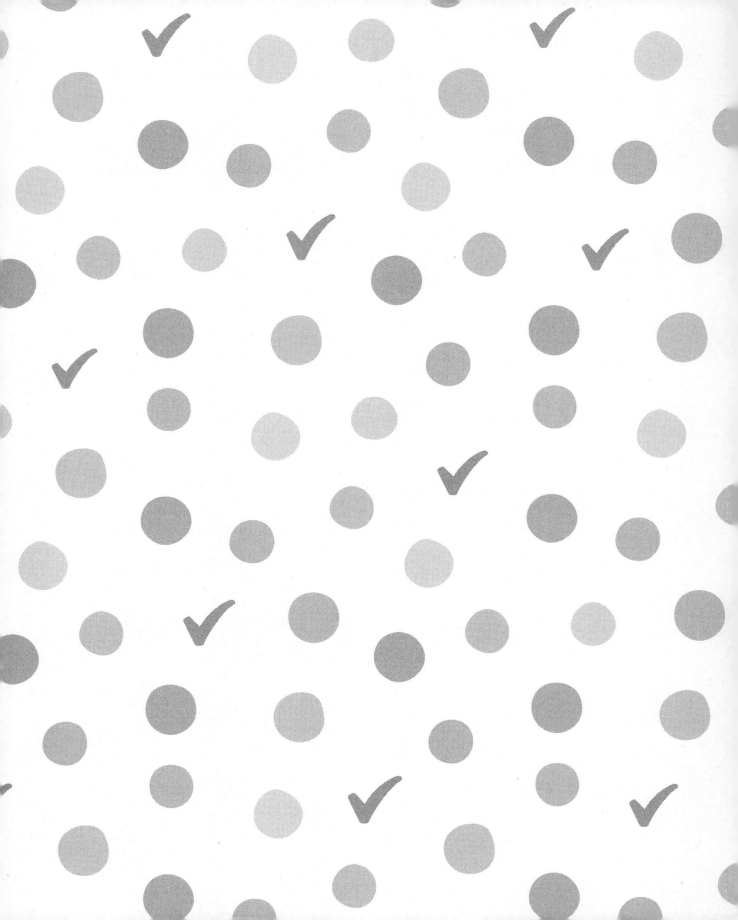

MENTAL HEALTH CHECKPOINT

Before a big adventure, it's good to take stock of what you have and what you need!

These questions can help. Answer them as honestly as you can.

What are three things going well in your life right now?

_____

_____

_____

_____

What are three things you're struggling with right now?

_____

_____

_____

_____

If you could change anything about your life, what would it be?

_____

_____

_____

_____

Who can you go to for help and support?

_____

_____

_____

_____

What would your closest friend say they like best about you?

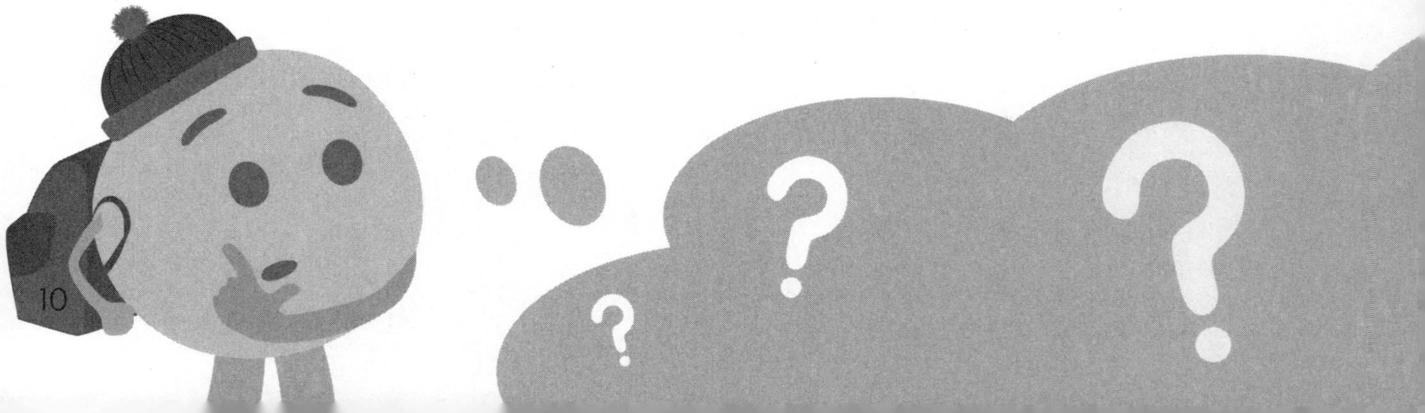

_____

_____

_____

_____

_____

What is your biggest fear for the future?

_____

_____

_____

_____

_____

What is your deepest hope or number one goal for the future?

_____

_____

_____

_____

_____

What is a challenge you've overcome in the past? How did you deal with it?

_____

_____

_____

_____

_____

WELLBEING AND HEALTH CHECK

People can feel good or not so good in areas of life ranging from physical and mental health to social life and relationships. Color in the box that best describes each area for you.

	EXCELLENT	GOOD	AVERAGE	POOR	VERY POOR
SLEEP					
FOOD/ EATING					
FRIENDSHIPS					
SCHOOL					
PHYSICAL HEALTH/MY BODY					
MENTAL HEALTH					
FAMILY LIFE					
HOBBIES/ PASSIONS					

Look at the boxes you filled in. Which areas do you need the most support with? What is hard for you in these areas?

_____

_____

_____

_____

Have you spoken to an adult you trust about your struggles in these areas? Put a "Y" for YES and an "N" for NO next to each area you could use support with.

If you wrote "Y" one or more times—that's great! Talking to a trusted adult about what's going on is an important step to figuring things out and getting help.

If you wrote "N" one or more times—that's okay. It can be hard to open up when you're struggling, but getting help or advice can be worth it.

Ask yourself:

- Would it be easiest to talk to an adult who knows you well, one who knows you somewhat, or one who doesn't know you at all, or only a little?
- Is there an adult you feel you could trust? This could be a family friend, a relative, or someone at your school.

If you don't know how to ask for help, you can use the help request card at the back of this book to start a conversation. If talking to someone you know feels too hard, start with an anonymous helpline for kids. To find a helpline in your area, search "Child Helpline International" online.

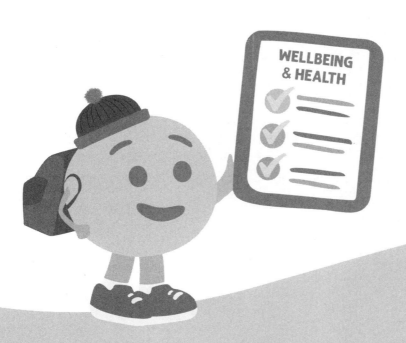

MINDSET CHECK

Three mindset ingredients will help on your journey: hope, willingness, and confidence. To check where you are with these as you start your journey, answer these questions as honestly as you can.

How **hopeful** are you that things can get better in the area(s) you chose above?

EXTREMELY **VERY** **SOMEWHAT** **A LITTLE** **NOT AT ALL**

How **willing** are you to learn new skills to help things get better?

EXTREMELY **VERY** **SOMEWHAT** **A LITTLE** **NOT AT ALL**

How **confident** are you in your ability to make change?

EXTREMELY **VERY** **SOMEWHAT** **A LITTLE** **NOT AT ALL**

If you're not feeling particularly hopeful, willing, or confident, why might that be?

For example, your brain might be telling you "I've tried things before and it didn't help" or "I don't believe things can change." These messages give you clues about your mindset.

Getting into the right mindset is key before a journey! Fortunately, each mindset ingredient is something you can build. The ideas below can help boost your hopefulness, willingness, and confidence. Put a star next to those you'll try.

Ideas to build **hope**:

- **KEEP WORKING ON YOUR VISION BOARD.** Include things you want for your life, even if they seem impossible (never-ending pizza machine, teleportation, a pet whale). The sky's the limit!

- **VISUALIZE A GOOD FUTURE.** Imagine yourself twenty years from now, living your dream life. See yourself free from things you're struggling with now. **What is it like?**

_____

_____

_____

_____

- **LOOK AT NATURE.** Things change constantly, and nature reminds us of this. Think of the weather, of leaves falling and growing back, of clouds shapeshifting in the wind. Everything changes, and the things you are struggling with will too.

Ideas to build **willingness**:

- **WRITE A PROS AND CONS LIST.** On one side of a piece of paper, list all the good things (pros) about trying something new (like a new skill from this book). On the other side, write any negative things (cons) about trying something new. Which side has a better argument?

- **THINK ABOUT HOW YOU COPE.** Do you try something, or watch and wait? Do you reach out, or keep it inside? Does your coping style work okay? Some ways of coping work in the short term but not so well over time. **What might happen if you keep coping with your problems the same way you are now, forever? What could be possible if you are willing to try a new way of coping?**

_____

_____

_____

_____

- **EXPERIMENT!** Great discoveries involve trying, learning from mistakes, and trying again. **Can you think of a time you tried something and it didn't work out, but you learned something or got there in the end?**

_____

_____

_____

_____

Life is full of moments like these—this might be one of them!

Ideas to build **confidence**:

- **CHECK IT OFF.** Write a list of everything you've done today—I mean **everything**—then check each item off. Got out of bed—check! Ate toast—check! Put a sock on my left foot—check! Put a sock on my right foot—check! You accomplish so many things every day. (These examples are small things, but even the biggest task can be broken down into small steps you can do!)
- **LOOK AT YOUR RECORD.** Remember some hard moments (or days) you've had. **Write a couple of words or draw a picture about a few of these.**

Not fun, right? But you made it through all that. That means your record for making it through is 100 percent! Now think about things you once didn't know how to do that are easy for you now—tying your shoes, using a knife and fork, riding a bike. Your brain has the amazing ability to learn: You've been doing it your whole life, and you'll go on to learn things you haven't even imagined yet.

- **FAKE IT TILL YOU MAKE IT.** Sometimes people need to give things a try, even without knowing how it will turn out. What would happen if you bravely tried the ideas in this book? (**HINT:** When people act confidently, over time they actually start *feeling* more confident....)

Now that you've taken stock, make a packing list of what you have and what you need.

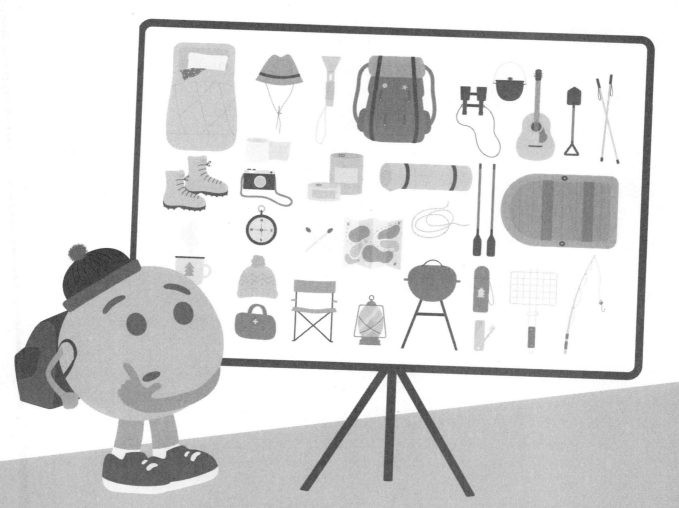

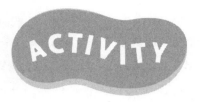

PACKING LIST

I ALREADY HAVE (for example, a sense of humor, kindness, math skills, family that loves me, the best cat):

_____

_____

_____

_____

_____

_____

_____

I STILL NEED (for example, more confidence, friendship skills, better sleep):

_____

_____

_____

_____

_____

_____

_____

Don't worry if there are things you need, or if you're not sure what you need—there are more ideas coming up, and you can add to both parts of the list as you go.

Chapter 3

TRAINING YOUR MIND AND BODY

Mountaineers spend years training their minds and bodies to handle the stresses of mountain climbing. This chapter will help you start your own mind and body training. Healthy habits will help you handle challenges now and in the future.

ABOUT YOUR BRAIN

Let's meet your brain (say "hello"...). It's pretty great. It's already learned a lot, and here it is, learning even more to help you have an amazing life. Let's talk about some cool things your brain can do!

Human brains have three main parts (there are lots more, but these are key). Your brain's in charge of:

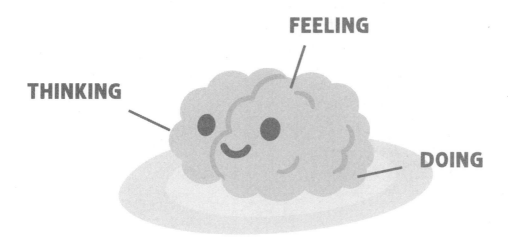

FEELING

THINKING

DOING

Your brain won't be fully grown until your late twenties. It's doing **a lot** of learning and growing. Right now, the parts of your brain in charge of feeling and doing are mostly running things. The thinking part is also busy, and will chime in more and more. As you get older, the parts of your brain will get better at talking to each other and working out what to do (rather than just reacting to whatever's happening).

One cool thing about your brain is that it is **flexible**. That means it can adapt to the world around you, figure out what's important, and solve problems creatively. This flexibility will help you navigate the ups and downs of life as you grow and have more experiences.

To understand how different parts of your brain handle information, think of a tricky moment from your week. What was happening in each part of your brain? (Imagine it if you can't remember.)

For example...

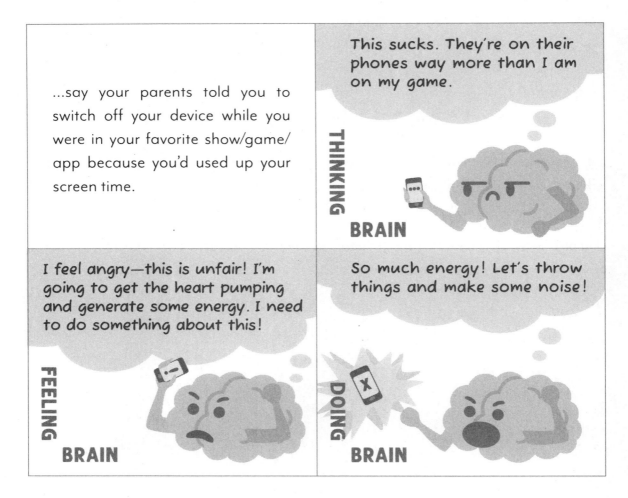

...say your parents told you to switch off your device while you were in your favorite show/game/app because you'd used up your screen time.

THINKING BRAIN

This sucks. They're on their phones way more than I am on my game.

FEELING BRAIN

I feel angry—this is unfair! I'm going to get the heart pumping and generate some energy. I need to do something about this!

DOING BRAIN

So much energy! Let's throw things and make some noise!

Now it's your turn. Below, write what happened during a tricky moment from your week. Then write what your thinking brain, feeling brain, and doing brain had to say about it.

	THINKING BRAIN
FEELING BRAIN	DOING BRAIN

What happens when your feeling brain is in charge of decision-making and you react in a big way? Does it make things better, or worse? What about when your doing brain is running things, and you react automatically, maybe without even realizing it?

Fortunately, you can learn more about how to use your brain's **flexibility** to manage tricky moments in more helpful ways. But first, let's talk about **practice**.

THE IMPORTANCE OF PRACTICE

If you really were about to trek up Mount Everest, it wouldn't be wise to just pack up and go without training beforehand. Similarly, it's important to train your body and mind for the challenges you could face in adolescence and beyond. Then, if you find yourself in a stressful situation, your training can kick in and help.

It's difficult for your brain to recall new information when you're stressed because it's busy trying to deal with the situation. Remember the three parts of your brain? When you're in a stressful situation, the thinking brain goes offline and the feeling and doing parts take over. If you've trained your brain to cope with stress, you'll be better able to stay cool and handle things.

All brains need repetition when learning something new. Think about how many times you had to practice tying your shoes before you mastered it. Practicing your new skills on small problems, and often, will help you use them more automatically with bigger problems. This is how you'll become a master of your mental health, by deciding to **practice** helpful skills until you become an expert at them.

At the end of this workbook (and at http://www.newharbinger.com/55633), you'll find a skill tracker like the one below. It will help you remember all the new tools you have in your pack. You can use it to track when you practice a new skill.

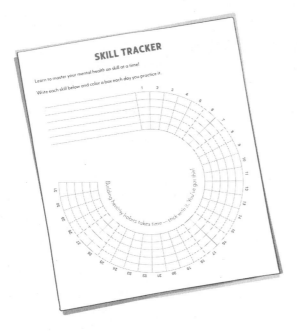

You'll see this symbol throughout the workbook to remind you to add a skill to your tracker:

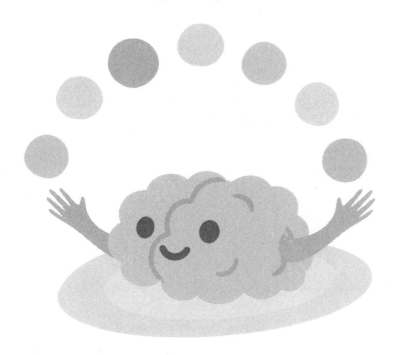

BONUS ACTIVITY To see just how quickly your brain can learn a skill with daily practice, try learning to juggle. It can be frustrating at the beginning, but if you practice at least five minutes every day, the movements start to feel automatic, and you'll keep the balls in the air even when distractions show up. Now, knowing how to juggle may not save your life one day, but the skills in this book might. Are you **willing** to practice the new skills in this book for at least five minutes a day?

AVOIDANCE IS OUT

Even when you really want to learn something new, it can be hard to stick to a routine and practice regularly. Sometimes we're so used to doing things one way that it's hard to change. Tricky thoughts, like doubts and fears, can talk you out of doing new things, even if they're good for you.

Do you ever put off doing new or difficult things, especially if you're not sure you can do them well? Let's play a quick game of "Never Do I Ever" to find out.

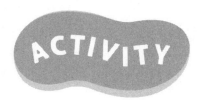

Circle the option that best describes you:

NEVER DO I EVER:

- Leave my homework to the last minute   **NEVER SOMETIMES ALWAYS**

- Speed-clean my room when someone is coming over   **NEVER SOMETIMES ALWAYS**

- Scroll on my phone or device to zone out   **NEVER SOMETIMES ALWAYS**

- Listen to music to drown out my thoughts   **NEVER SOMETIMES ALWAYS**

- Turn down an opportunity to try something because I might be bad at it or embarrass myself   **NEVER SOMETIMES ALWAYS**

- Say yes to things to avoid conflict or keep other people happy   **NEVER SOMETIMES ALWAYS**

- Distract myself when big emotions show up   **NEVER SOMETIMES ALWAYS**

- Withdraw from people when I'm feeling anxious or sad   **NEVER SOMETIMES ALWAYS**

- Spend hours gaming/reading/scrolling to avoid real life   **NEVER SOMETIMES ALWAYS**

- Think about things on repeat, way more times than I need to   **NEVER SOMETIMES ALWAYS**

All brains are built to avoid pain, discomfort, and danger. So it's totally normal that your brain has found clever ways of coping when things are tough. But here's the thing: Avoidance only works in the short term. The problems, thoughts, and feelings you are avoiding today are just being pushed aside. They'll be right there waiting for you tomorrow. When you keep using old habits or avoidance to cope, the problems build up and then explode out.

The next activity will help you discover if the coping strategies you're using are really helping you in the long term.

What thoughts, feelings, memories, or situations do you wish you could get rid of forever?

_____

_____

_____

_____

_____

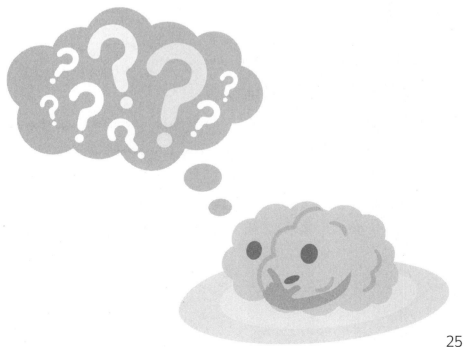

In the table, mark the things you've done to try to avoid, ignore, or get rid of those thoughts, feelings, memories, or situations. If there are other things you've tried, write them in the "other" column.

DISTRACTING	OPTING OUT	THINKING	OTHER
Watching TV/movies/ YouTube	Leaving early	Worrying	Eating or drinking
Listening to music	Not going to school	Dwelling on the past	Using substances
Reading	Staying in my room	Daydreaming	
Scrolling	Turning down an invitation	Planning out the future	
Exercise	Not taking a new opportunity	Imagining ways to escape	
Self-harm	Saying "I don't care" when I do care	Trying to only "look on the bright side"	
Helping others	Keeping away from things that trigger anxiety	Blaming others	
Cleaning/organizing/ rearranging	Hiding the real me to fit in	Criticizing myself	

Thinking about each of the things on the list that you marked, answer these two questions:

1. Did this get rid of your difficult thoughts/feelings/memories forever, or keep them from coming back? **YES / NO**

2. Did this help you become more like the person you want to be, or have the life you want to live? **YES / NO**

WHAT TO DO INSTEAD

Avoiding problems may have helped in the moment. But it probably hasn't helped you in the long run. It may have even made things worse or meant you missed out on some great things. You may have acted in ways you regret. Or maybe it's too tiring to keep up. So let's not do that anymore. Avoidance is out, acceptance is in. Acceptance means getting okay with how things are—even if you don't like or want them.

Here's the first tool to add to your pack. It's a saying to help you remember that avoidance only helps in the short term. And you're learning skills for the long haul. To overcome challenges, you need to:

NAME IT TO TAME IT

FEEL IT TO HEAL IT

This means you need to face difficult things that are happening. And you need to feel the feelings that show up. Don't bottle feelings up, distract yourself, or push feelings away. Acceptance means letting things be what they are, without trying to change them.

(Later, you'll learn how to help yourself when the feelings are uncomfortable or you have to accept things you don't like or can't change. So read on!)

Color in the poster on the next page while you let this new idea sink in.

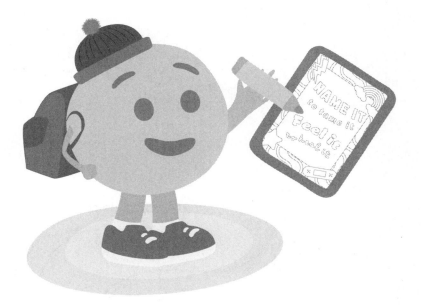

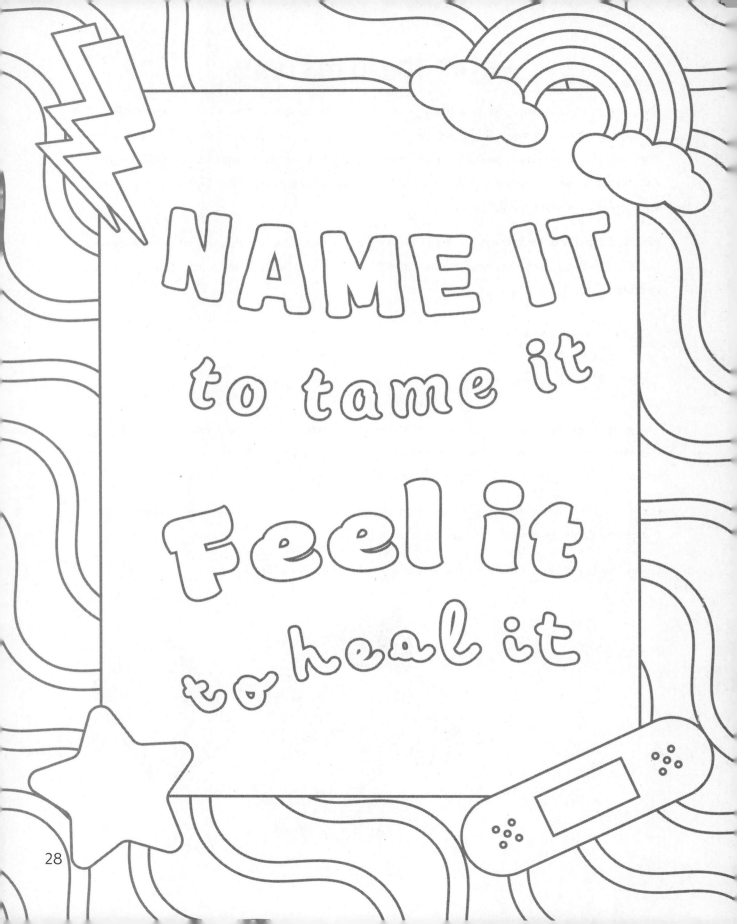

NAME IT
to tame it
Feel it
to heal it

28

TAKE CARE OF YOUR BODY TO HELP YOUR MIND

Your physical health and mental health are connected. This means taking care of your body is an important part of being healthy and well.

GET THOSE ZZZS

There's no way around it—you need sleep to survive! During sleep, your brain and body repair themselves. You are growing, sorting information, processing memories, and recovering from the day. Not getting enough sleep makes it really hard for your brain and body to work properly. It can lead to serious mental and physical health problems.

Use the sleep tracker below to record what your sleep is like now. This will help you know if you have sleep problems, or are not getting enough sleep. You need 8 to 9 hours of good sleep every night—more if you're sick, having a growth spurt, or feeling run down.

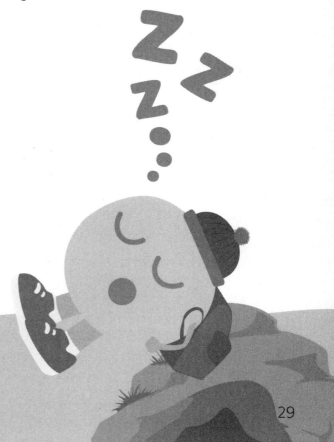

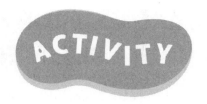

SLEEP TRACKER

DAY	TIME I WENT TO SLEEP LAST NIGHT	TIME I WOKE UP THIS MORNING	TOTAL HOURS OF SLEEP	I HAD TROUBLE FALLING ASLEEP (YES / NO)	I HAD TROUBLE STAYING ASLEEP (YES / NO)	I WOKE UP FEEL-ING WELL RESTED (YES / NO)

Here are some ways to hack your sleep to get a better night's rest.

KEEP BED FOR SLEEPING Don't read or watch shows in bed. When your head hits that pillow at night, your brain needs to know it's time to sleep. When you do other things in bed, your brain learns it's another place to be alert and awake—the opposite of what you want. This also means no daytime naps—save all those ZZZs for bedtime and your bed.

GET REGULAR Brains love routine, so going to bed and waking up at the same time every day means a happier brain. The closer you stick to your sleep routine, the easier it will be to fall asleep and wake up at those times. If summer vacation has its own, different routine, that's okay. Just try to get back into your school sleep routine a week or two before school starts.

USE SLEEP RITUALS Did your parents have a sleep ritual for you when you were little? Maybe you enjoyed a bath before bed or reading stories together. Maybe you had a special light on or a relaxing smell in your room, like lavender. You may have outgrown your nightlight (or not, it's all good), but your brain will still enjoy a little ritual before bed. Maybe drink a warm milk drink, take a warm bath or shower, do some gentle stretching, color or write in a journal, dim the lights, or listen to soft music. What would feel soothing and relaxing for you before you head off to dreamland? (No screens: They can keep you awake long after you've turned them off!)

MAKE THE SPACE RIGHT Your bedroom is your special place. Getting it just right for sleep—quiet, dark, and not too hot or too cold—can make a big difference. It should feel safe. Talk to your parents: What changes can you make to your room to help you sleep?

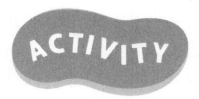

YOUR SLEEP ROUTINE

Think about your sleep routine. Give yourself 5 points for each of the good sleep hacks you already use.

I only use my bed for sleeping. _____ *points*

I don't take naps during the day. _____ *points*

I go to bed and wake up around the same time every day. _____ *points*

I have a bedtime routine that helps me relax. _____ *points*

I don't look at screens for an hour before bedtime. _____ *points*

My bedroom is safe and comfortable. _____ *points*

Total score _____ */ 30 points*

What new sleep hack can you use to get a better night's rest? Try it for a week or two. Then do the sleep tracker again to see what's changed.

NOURISH YOUR BRAIN AND BODY

Eating regularly and having a wide range of foods helps fuel your brain and body. No one made it to the top of Mount Everest on a few rice crackers! You may not be in charge of buying the food or cooking the meals in your house, so here are the general rules:

1. Make the most of the food you have available.

2. Be willing to try new things.

3. Eat regularly (every three to four hours while you're awake).

4. Stay hydrated by drinking plenty of water.

Food is tricky for some people. Maybe you use it to distract yourself. Or maybe you find it hard to eat at times. Remember that food is fuel, and every human body needs fuel to survive. As best you can, give your body good fuel to help it grow and be healthy.

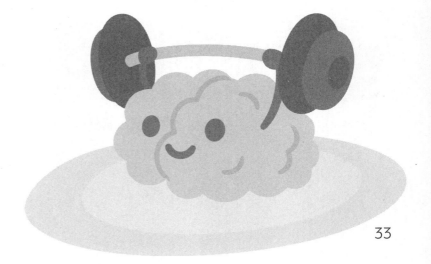

If you were going to fuel your body for a big adventure, what foods would you choose? List them here, or draw pictures (or both!).

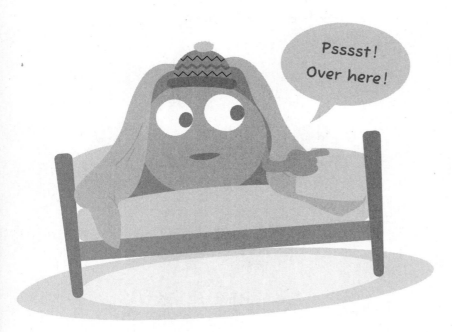

Pssssst! Over here!

If you struggle with food and eating, body image, or controlling your food or body size, it's super important to let a trusted adult know. The information in this workbook will still be helpful, but you may need some extra support. In the back of this workbook is a help request card you can fill out and give to an adult you trust.

KEEP MOVING!

Moving your body helps keep your muscles and joints strong. It also helps you manage your emotions and keep your brain healthy. If you already do something active—a sport, dancing, walking your dog—great! If not, use the ideas below to add more movement to your day. Put a star next to the idea you like the best. Then add it to your skill tracker to remind you to do it every day!

- **DANCE IT OUT.** Put on your favorite music and have your own personal dance party. This can be a great mood booster!

- **STRETCH IT OUT.** Wake your body up or wind it down with some gentle stretching. Search "yoga for middle-schoolers" online or try the yoga poses shown on the next page. Yoga is great for both body and mind, and can help you feel more relaxed.

- **LIFT IT.** Find some weights around the house: canned food, filled water bottles, a full laundry basket, or your own body weight (like doing push-ups) all work. Lifting weight can help you release energy and lower stress or anxiety.

- **GET YOUR HEART RATE UP.** Find a jump rope, do some jumping jacks, or run down the street and back. Raising your heart rate increases the "feel-good" chemicals in your brain and can help you get through a rough day.

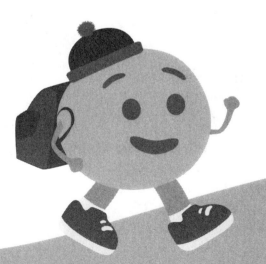

YOGA POSES

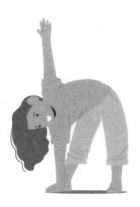

TRIANGLE

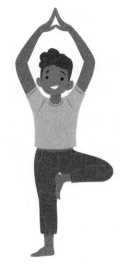

TREE

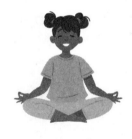

LOTUS

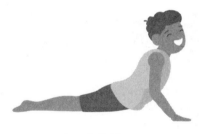

COBRA

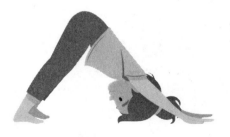

DOWNWARD DOG

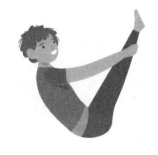

BOAT

SELF-CARE

When life gets tough, good daily habits can start to slip. You can get stuck in a cycle of feeling bad, then not taking good care of yourself, then feeling worse. Good personal care can help you get back on track.

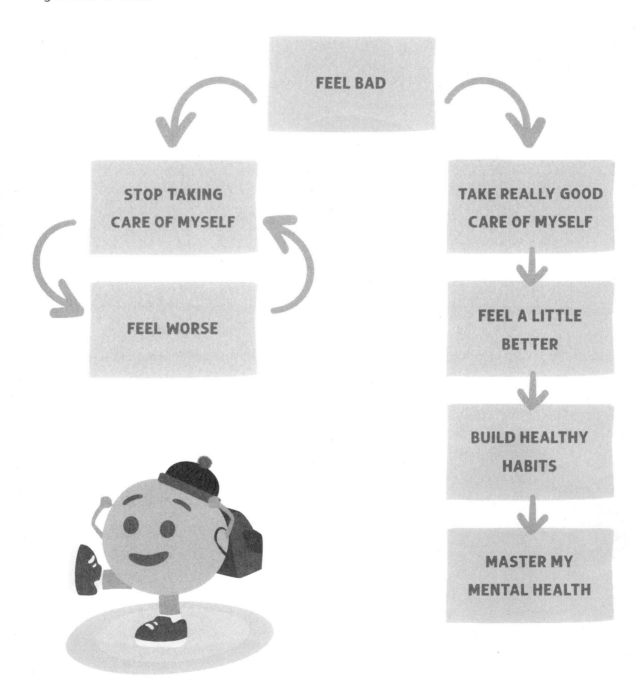

Use this checklist as a gentle daily reminder to take care of yourself. Snap a photo of the list or copy it, and stick it somewhere in your room to help you remember.

Daily Checklist

Have I:

- ☐ Showered
- ☐ Brushed my teeth
- ☐ Washed my face
- ☐ Brushed my hair
- ☐ Put on clean clothes
- ☐ Put on deodorant
- ☐ Taken my medication (if needed)
- ☐ _____
- ☐ _____

Good self-care also means getting medical help when you need it. If something isn't feeling right, or an illness or injury isn't getting better over time, ask a trusted adult to help you.

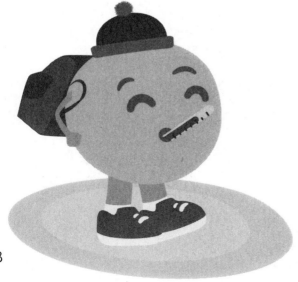

YOUR WELLNESS PLAN

Make a promise to yourself to take the best possible care you can of your brain and body, so you can keep climbing all the way to the top! Fill out the wellness plan below. You may want to look at the wellbeing and health check you did in Chapter 1. Which areas are going well? What needs your attention?

My body is my home. I will take good care of it by:

Things I will do more of (for example, going to bed at the same time each night, drinking plenty of water, brushing my teeth every day):

Things I will do less of (for example, skipping meals, being on screens close to bedtime, doing things to avoid difficult thoughts):

Don't forget to add skills to your tracker at the back of the book!

Don't forget to add skills to your tracker at the back of the book!

BONUS TIP Share your health plan with the people you live with, close friends, or a trusted adult. People who care about you can support you on your journey—like a personal cheer squad.

You've learned a lot in this chapter about training your mind and body to handle stress in healthy ways and keep you moving toward an awesome life. If you plan to try ideas from this chapter, pause here and give yourself a week or two to build those healthy habits before moving to the next chapter. Skills take time to build, and supporting your mental health is worth it!

BECOMING WISE AND KIND

Welcome to the next part of the journey—becoming wise and kind! In this chapter, you'll learn about mindfulness and self-compassion. These super-strengths can help you live life to the fullest and get through tough times.

MINDFULNESS: NOTICING THE NOW

Can you remember the last time you brushed your teeth or put socks on? If you can't, it's probably because you were on autopilot—doing things without thinking. When you do things often, your brain stops paying close attention to what you're doing. Your autopilot takes over. This can be helpful (imagine if you had to tell yourself to breathe before every single breath!).

But when your **doing brain** is on autopilot, your **thinking brain** might start worrying about the future or dwelling on the past. When that happens, you are no longer living **in the now**. The solution for this is **mindfulness**.

Mindfulness is the skill of **noticing** and being **curious** about what is happening right here and now. When you are mindful, you are living in the present. You notice more of what is going on around you *and* inside of you.

This matters because when you notice more, you can choose what you want to focus on and what you want to do. Mindfulness can help **you** be in control of your life. It helps you pause and choose how you want to **respond** to what is happening instead of reacting without thinking.

Here's a quick experiment. Stop reading for a moment and notice:

5 THINGS YOU CAN SEE

4 THINGS YOU CAN TOUCH

3 THINGS YOU CAN HEAR

2 THINGS YOU CAN SMELL

1 THING YOU CAN TASTE

What happened while you were noticing these things? Was your mind thinking about anything else? How do you feel after paying close attention to the things around you?

Being mindful can mean you notice **more** of what's going on. You might notice sounds in the distance. You might feel or enjoy your experiences more, for example really noticing the taste and texture of food while eating.

Imagine being on autopilot during a mountain-climbing adventure. What details might you miss?

Are there ways you get stuck on autopilot that make your current situation worse? (For example, thinking too much about the past, unhelpful habits, reacting rather than responding.)

When things aren't going well in life, your mind can get stuck in a negative loop. It may only notice things that are going wrong, focus on difficult thoughts or feelings, or make up stories (worries) about bad things that could happen in the future. Mindfulness can help you notice when you're stuck in a negative loop and focus on other things that are going on around you.

What do you think would happen if you were more mindful and got curious about what is happening around you and inside of you? How might that help you with the struggles you're facing?

Can you find the eight hiking symbols in the image? Cross them out as you find them.

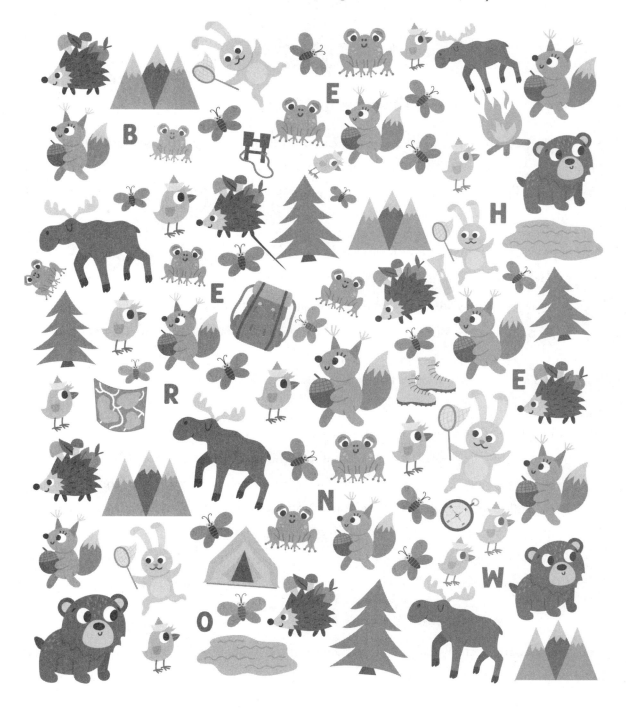

Did you notice the hidden message in the picture? Sometimes it helps to slow down and get curious....

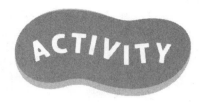

STAYING CURIOUS

Has your brain ever jumped to the wrong conclusion? Mindfulness can help with that. Mindfulness means staying curious about what you notice, not labeling or judging it. This helps you notice what is **actually** happening, and not get lost in the stories your brain tells you about what **could** happen.

Try this activity to see how your brain likes to label and judge.

1. Take out a piece of paper and something to draw with.

2. Draw a squiggly line or design that takes up the whole page.

3. Sit back, look at your drawing, and notice what your thinking brain has to say about it—do judgmental thoughts show up, like: "That's not good"; "I can't draw"; or "This is dumb"? Was your brain thinking about other things while you were drawing? If so, just notice them.

4. Pause and take a few slow, deep breaths.

5. Retrace the line; this time, imagine this is your first time holding a pen or pencil. Retrace **slowly**, paying attention to the feel of the pen or pencil in your hands, what it feels like as it moves across the paper. Notice any changes in color or shading. Stay **curious** about the experience and what you might notice.

6. What happened to your thoughts when you slowed down and focused more on what was happening in the moment? Did you feel any different when you were more mindful and less judgmental?

You can repeat this activity. Stay curious about what you might notice. Check in with how you feel after a few moments of being more present.

Think about something you're struggling with now, or a time when you made a mistake. Write down any unkind words or judgments your brain made about **you**.

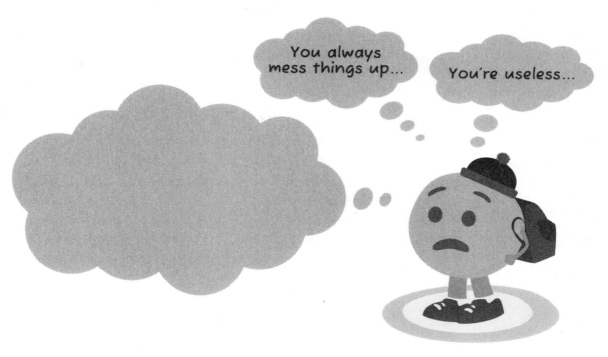

How does it feel to look at those unkind words?

SELF-COMPASSION: BEING KIND TO YOURSELF

Everyone has an unkind voice in their mind, and everyone goes through tough times. That's why self-compassion is so important! Self-compassion means being kind to yourself, especially when things are tough.

Look at the unkind words you wrote about yourself on page 47. Imagine your closest friend was saying those things about themself. What would you say or do to comfort them?

Most people find it easier to be kind to others than to themselves. To be kind to yourself:

1. Notice what's going on for you (using mindfulness).

2. Offer yourself kindness (just like you would offer a friend).

3. Remember you're not alone (everyone goes through tough times).

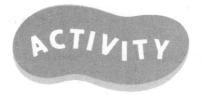

COMPASSIONATE LETTER

Write yourself a compassionate letter to find your compassionate voice.

1. Find a quiet space. Think about something challenging you've been through.

2. Write a letter to yourself, like you're your own best friend.

3. Be kind and supportive. What would a good friend write to comfort and encourage you?

4. Read your letter and notice how you feel.

MINDFUL MOMENTS JOURNAL

Your preteen years will be full of special moments, big and small. A Mindful Moments Journal helps you capture them. This can remind you that even on tough days, there are glimmers of fun, joy, and things to be grateful for. For your journal, you can use a notebook, a memo or journal app, or whatever paper comes to hand. Then:

1. Throughout the day, pause and notice moments when you feel happy, calm, or curious.

2. Write a few words or draw a picture to remember each moment you notice.

3. You can write a little about what it's like to notice these small moments. Do you feel happy? Grateful? Surprised?

4. Before bed, look back at your mindful moments from the day. How do you feel looking back at them?

BONUS CHALLENGE Share your mindful moments with a friend or family member. Ask them about details they noticed in their day. How does it feel to share these moments?

Remember, becoming wise and kind is like training your mind muscles. You're building mental strength and flexibility, which will help you as you keep climbing. The more you practice, the easier it gets.

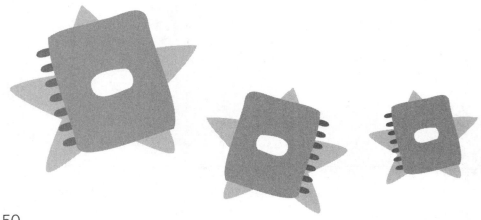

Here are some ideas for incorporating more mindfulness and self-compassion into your day.

- **TAKE A MENTAL PHOTO:** Pause and take a mental snapshot of what's in front of you. Try to notice as many details as you can about what you see, hear, feel, and smell.

- **PLANT SEEDS OF KINDNESS:** Do a random act of kindness for someone; notice how you feel.

- **CATCH YOUR BREATH:** Take a slow breath in, hold for one second, then slowly breathe out through your mouth as if you're blowing through a straw. Notice all the little movements that happen in your body as you breathe.

- **FIND YOUR FEET:** Push your feet into the floor (you can sit or stand while you do this) and notice the feeling of your muscles working and the ground supporting you.

- **MIRROR, MIRROR:** Look in the mirror and say one kind thing to yourself.

- **SAY THANKS:** Express your gratitude for one thing every day, big or small.

- **A KIND GESTURE:** Give yourself support by putting a hand over your heart, hugging yourself, or holding your own hand. This can help you remind yourself that you're learning to treat yourself with kindness when things are tough.

In the list above, circle two ideas you're going to try this week and add them to your skill tracker.

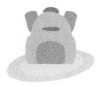 Slowing down, staying curious, and noticing more of what is happening right now will help you make better decisions. It will also help you be more present on your journey through middle school. Supporting yourself with kindness when things are hard helps you overcome the challenges you're facing, without making yourself feel worse.

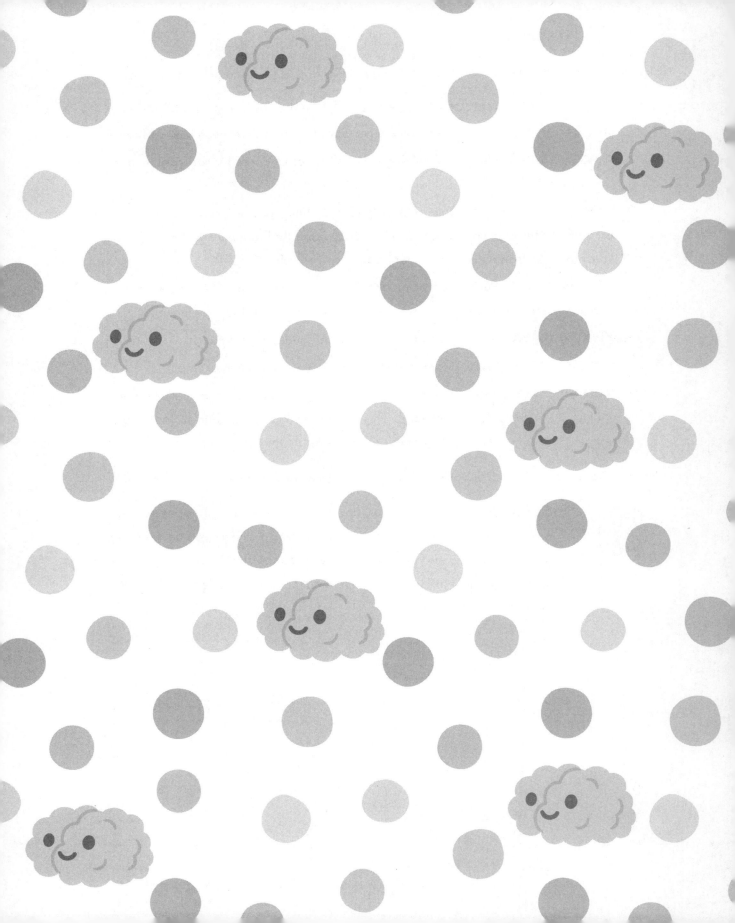

Chapter 5

MASTERING YOUR THOUGHTS

In this chapter, we'll ask some questions about the thinking part of your brain:

WHAT ARE THOUGHTS?

WHERE DO THEY COME FROM?

ARE THEY ALWAYS TRUE?

CAN YOU CONTROL YOUR THOUGHTS?

As we think about thoughts, you'll practice using the skill of mindfulness to **notice what's going on inside your mind**. It's the first step to making good decisions about what to do.

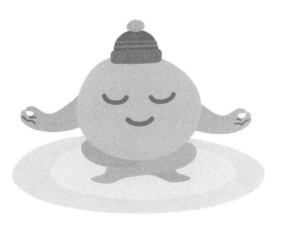

FIXED VERSUS FLEXIBLE THOUGHTS

In Chapter 3, you learned your brain is **flexible**—it can keep changing throughout your life.

When life is challenging, your brain saves energy by thinking and doing things in the same way over and over. Sometimes, our brains can get stuck on the same idea or way of doing things. This can make it harder to find creative solutions to problems or try new things. Another word for "stuck" is **fixed,** which describes something that won't or can't change. So "fixed" is the opposite of "flexible."

Look around you and write down three things you can see that are fixed—**that can't or don't move or change:**

_____

_____

_____

Now write down three things you can see that are flexible—**that can move or change:**

_____

_____

_____

When your thoughts become fixed, you're more likely to give up. Fixed thoughts about yourself or your situation often sound like this:

I don't know how to_____.   I can't do it.

This won't work.   I'll never be able to_____.

I don't understand_____.   I don't get it.

I'm not good at this.

How do you feel when you read that list? Do those thoughts help you feel hopeful, like things could get better, or that you could improve? Probably not!

You can change a fixed mindset with just one small word. **Can you guess what it is?**

_____   _____   _____

Go back and add "yet" to each of the fixed mindset sentences above. What changes? Could adding "yet" help you to feel more hopeful that things could change?

Having a fixed mindset is like a big rock blocking your path—it's hard to move past. But if your path was blocked with snow instead, you could make a way through, moving or melting it.

Use your flexible brain to find a way through this maze:

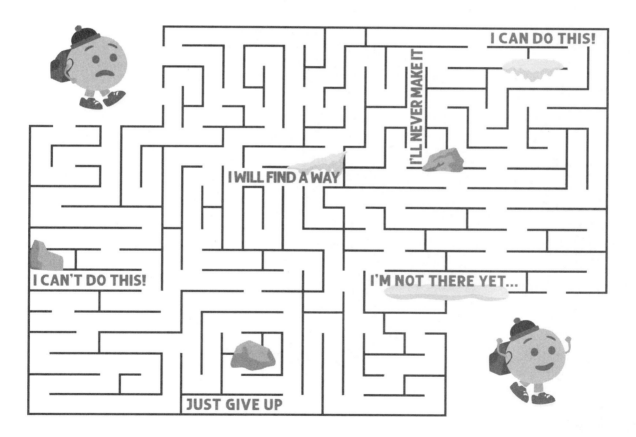

You can learn anything. **You can** improve at anything you put time and effort into practicing. That includes getting better at mastering your thoughts and feelings, and overcoming things you're struggling with.

EXPLORING YOUR MENTAL LANDSCAPE

Your brain is an amazing thinking machine. Some thoughts are really helpful and some are very unhelpful (most are somewhere in the middle). In the next few pages, you'll learn how to notice your thoughts as they happen, and decide whether they are helpful or not.

NOTICING THOUGHTS

For the next sixty seconds, think of a problem you're facing. Then write about or draw a picture of everything that went through your mind about the situation in that one minute.

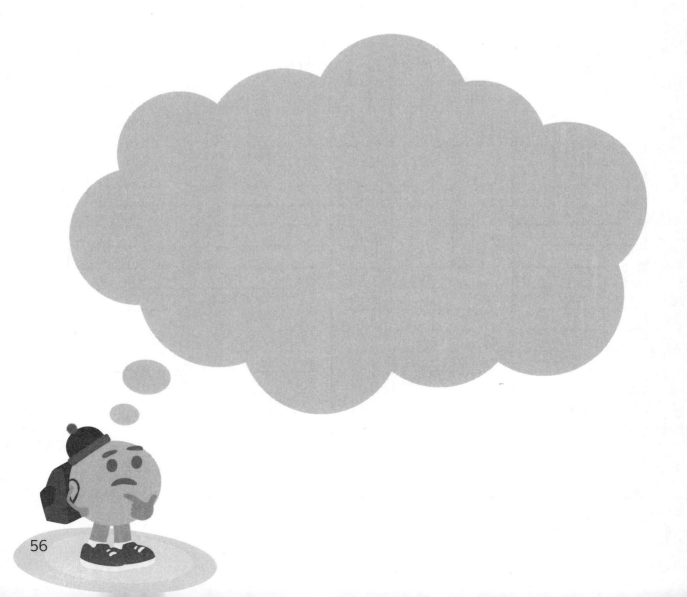

Your brain thinks thousands of thoughts every day. Some are random, some deep and meaningful. Sometimes you'll be thinking about something in particular (like what's for dinner, or something your friend said yesterday). Sometimes your mind will play: It might count things, replay songs, or imagine what you'll do this weekend. It's normal to have lots of thoughts, and for some of them to be random!

Look at the thoughts you wrote down above. How many are positive? How many are negative, neutral, or just random? Choose three different colored pencils or markers to circle the **positive**, **negative**, and **neutral** (or random) thoughts. Which color occurs the most?

Remember your brain likes repetition. It forms habits out of the things you do most often. So if your brain spends a lot of time thinking negative thoughts, it can become harder for you to see the positive and neutral things in your life. It's like wearing doom and gloom glasses—everything you look at through them seems negative, even if it's not.

If you'd like to help your thoughts be more balanced, start a **highlight of my day** jar. In it, save reminders of positive or neutral things from your day (either written on a slip of paper, or a souvenir of a good event). You could also use a gratitude journal: a notebook where you record things you're grateful for. Over time, your brain will start to hunt for positive moments and pay less attention to negative ones.

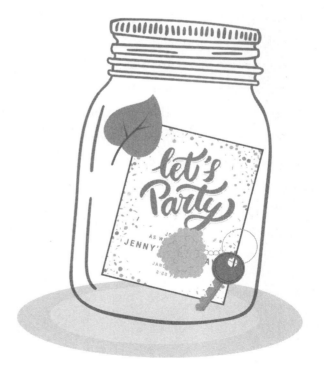

THINKING RUTS

When you're facing a problem, the thinking part of your brain gets busy looking for solutions. **Think about a problem you're facing. Take a few minutes to write down all the solutions your thinking brain has come up with.**

The problem:

_____

_____

My solutions:

_____

_____

_____

_____

Your brain is always **trying** to help you. But when things in life are really difficult and there are no clear or quick solutions to your problems, it can get stuck. Sometimes it gets in **thinking ruts**, either stuck thinking about things from your past (this is called ruminating) or stuck imagining things about the future (this is called worrying). Imagine finding what looked like a shortcut to the top of the mountain, only to discover it's a dead end, or took you way off course. Thinking ruts can be like that—they might seem familiar, or like they will help, but they usually make things worse in the long run.

Check out the thinking ruts below and color in the ones your brain has tried:

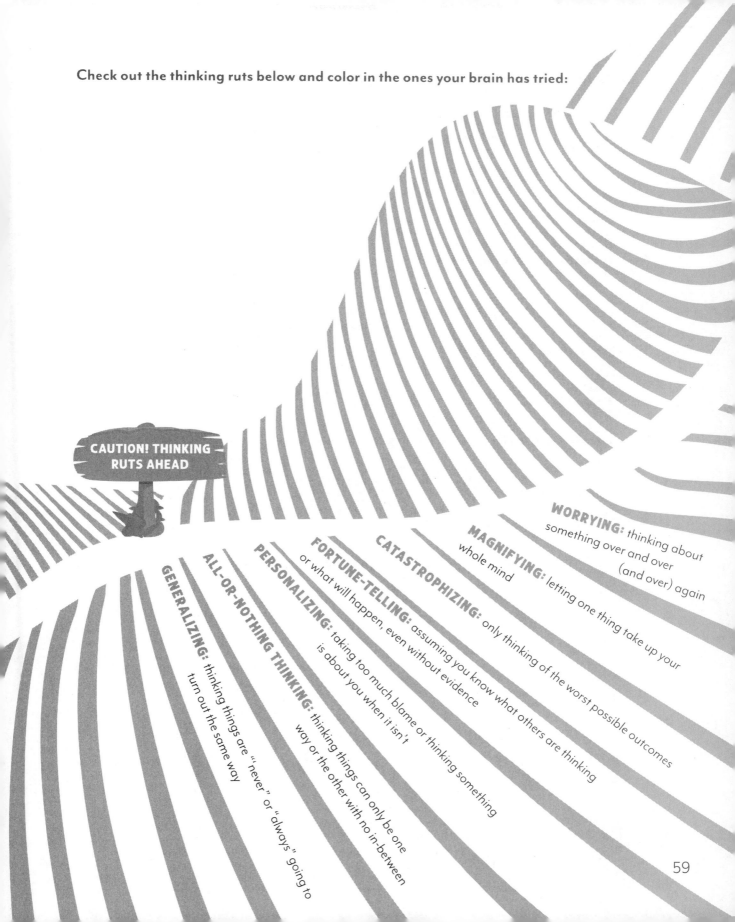

CAUTION! THINKING RUTS AHEAD

WORRYING: thinking about something over and over (and over) again

MAGNIFYING: letting one thing take up your whole mind

CATASTROPHIZING: only thinking of the worst possible outcomes

FORTUNE-TELLING: assuming you know what others are thinking or what will happen, even without evidence

PERSONALIZING: taking too much blame or thinking something is about you when it isn't

ALL-OR-NOTHING THINKING: thinking things can only be one way or the other with no in-between

GENERALIZING: thinking things are "never" or "always" going to turn out the same way

Write down a time when your brain got stuck in a thinking rut. What was happening?

_____

_____

_____

_____

What thoughts were going through your mind?

_____

_____

_____

_____

One way to get yourself back on track is to ask yourself three questions about the thought:

1. **IS IT TRUE?**

2. **IS IT HELPFUL?**

3. **IS IT KIND?**

The kinds of thoughts brains can get stuck on usually have at least one "no" answer to these questions.

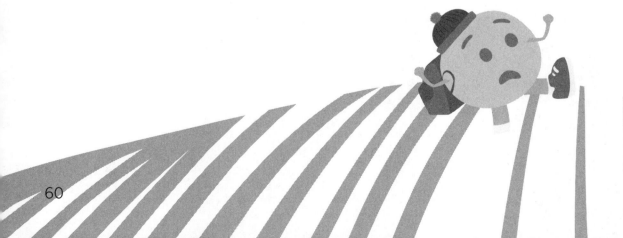

Specifically, some thoughts might be true, but not helpful or kind. For example, if your friends ran off at lunchtime and you think "everyone has left me," that part may be true. But your brain probably doesn't stop there. Instead, it adds thoughts like: "they must all hate me" (fortune-telling); "I'll never have any real friends" (generalizing); or "I'm a loser" (personalizing). Those quickly turn into thinking ruts, and they're not true, helpful, or kind.

In this example, a more true, helpful, kind thought is: "Oh, my friends ran off. I wonder what happened? I'll ask when I see them next."

Look at the thoughts you wrote down about the time your brain got stuck in a thinking rut. Are any of those thoughts untrue, unhelpful, or unkind? Can you change any of them to be more true, helpful, and kind?

A more true, helpful, or kind thought is:

_____

_____

_____

_____

_____

Now that you know about thinking ruts, you can look out for them. Remember: They may seem true because they feel familiar, or they may look like shortcuts, but they don't help you in the long run!

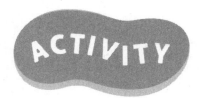

THOUGHTS ARE NOT FACTS EXPERIMENT

Let's do an experiment to help you remember that not all thoughts are true.

Think to yourself, as convincingly as you can—I AM A DUCK!

Repeat the thought over and over in your mind. Say it out loud if you want to, and notice what happens...

Anything...?

Did you suddenly sprout feathers? Have an urge to jump in a pond? Quack out loud?

No?

That's because simply thinking something doesn't make it true. The thought doesn't have any power of its own: It's just a thought.

But what happens when you think something negative about yourself? Let's test that.

Pick one of the judgmental thoughts you wrote on page 47 and repeat it over and over in your mind—I'm dumb, everyone hates me, it's all my fault. Notice what happens.

It might **feel** true, and it probably doesn't feel very nice. But remember, simply thinking something doesn't make it true. If thinking "I'm a duck" doesn't make you a duck, then thinking "I'm a bad kid" doesn't make you a bad kid. (Also, "I'm a bad kid" is not kind **or** helpful: That's another clue your brain is getting off track.) You are not your thoughts, and your thoughts don't have power unless you act on them!

GETTING THOUGHTS BACK ON TRACK

What can you do when untrue, unhelpful, or unkind thoughts are taking you off track?

Below, write things that are important to you or that you want to learn, try, or improve at. Then write down the untrue, unhelpful, or unkind thoughts that show up and take you off track. (Following the unhelpful thoughts is going to take you **away** from the life you want.) Add some true, helpful, kind thoughts to help you stay on track and move **toward** the life you want.

THINGS THAT MATTER TO ME	THOUGHTS THAT TAKE ME OFF TRACK	THOUGHTS THAT HELP ME STAY ON TRACK

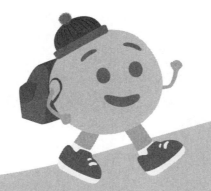

HAPPY HEALTHY ADULT SUMMIT

Things will never change.

It's too hard.

What if...

I can't cope with this.

It's all my fault.

There's no point trying.

This is important to me.

I believe in myself.

I can ask for help.

I'm still learning.

I can do hard things.

Small steps are still steps.

64

You can't stop your brain thinking and you've already learned that avoiding difficult thoughts and feelings doesn't help in the long run. You might **have** difficult thoughts (your thinking brain makes them up), but **you** are not your thoughts. That means **you can choose** how to act and what to do, even when unhelpful thoughts show up and try to take you off track.

Still not convinced? Think to yourself—"I can't stand up" (or another simple movement). Really tell yourself it's true.

Now, stand up!

You can choose to do so many things, even if your thoughts are telling you otherwise.

Separating yourself from your thoughts gives you space. In that space you can make a wise, kind choice about what you want to do, based on what is most important to you. Here are ways to help you step back from your thoughts:

- **USE THE "IS IT TRUE/HELPFUL/KIND" QUESTIONS ON PAGE 60.** If any of the answers is "no," simply thank your brain for its suggestion. Then do something that's important or that you enjoy.

- **ASK "IS IT SOLVABLE?"** Some questions can't be answered **yet**, some problems can't be solved **yet**, and no amount of thinking, talking, researching, or worrying will change that. If you realize something can't be solved yet, focus on something you **can** do right now (more about this in the next chapter).

- **SEND IT DOWN THE MOUNTAIN.** Imagine writing each fixed or unhelpful thought on a rock and watching it roll down the mountain and away. Those thoughts can stay down there. Your goals are taking you onward and upward!

- **QUACK LIKE A DUCK.** Imagine the thoughts are being quacked at you by a tiny duck in your mind. Sounds ridiculous? Good! You're not going to take anything that duck says too seriously because thoughts are not facts, and you are not your thoughts. Have a little laugh at your inner thought duck and get back on track.

What about the really tough, painful thoughts and feelings?

When your brain is tired, scared, sad, or overwhelmed, it can't think of good solutions to problems. When your brain runs out of good ideas, you might think the best solution is to avoid, retreat, or hide as much as you can. This can be scary and lonely, and it means you need help. Things **can**
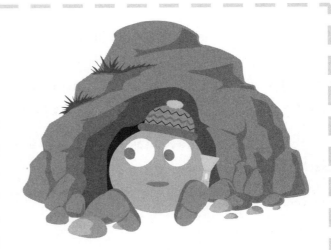
change—in fact, it's almost guaranteed they will. If you're having a lot of painful thoughts and feelings, use the help request card at the end of this book. Give it to a trusted adult to let them know your brain has run out of ideas to solve your problem and you need help.

Let's tie some things together.

MINDFULNESS
FLEXIBILITY
SELF-COMPASSION

You can use the skill of **mindfulness** to notice your thoughts. This will help you notice unhelpful thoughts and thinking ruts. You can use your brain's **flexibility** to practice new skills, find creative solutions, and move toward the life you want. When your mind is being unkind or life's challenges are causing you pain, use **self-compassion to give yourself comfort and support.**

Choose a tool from this chapter to add to your skill tracker at the end of this book. Then use the poster on page 68 to write a saying that will help you remember that tool or skill.

Here are some examples:

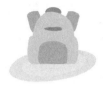

- I'm not a duck, and thoughts aren't facts.

- I'm not there YET.

- I am not my thoughts.

- Is what I'm thinking true, helpful, or kind?

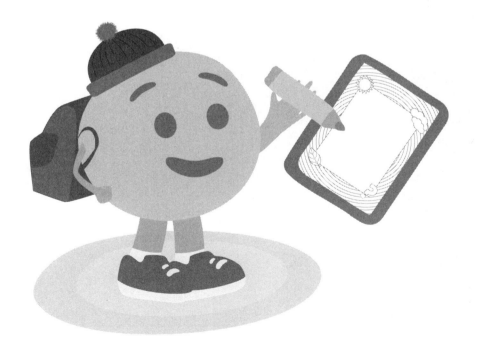

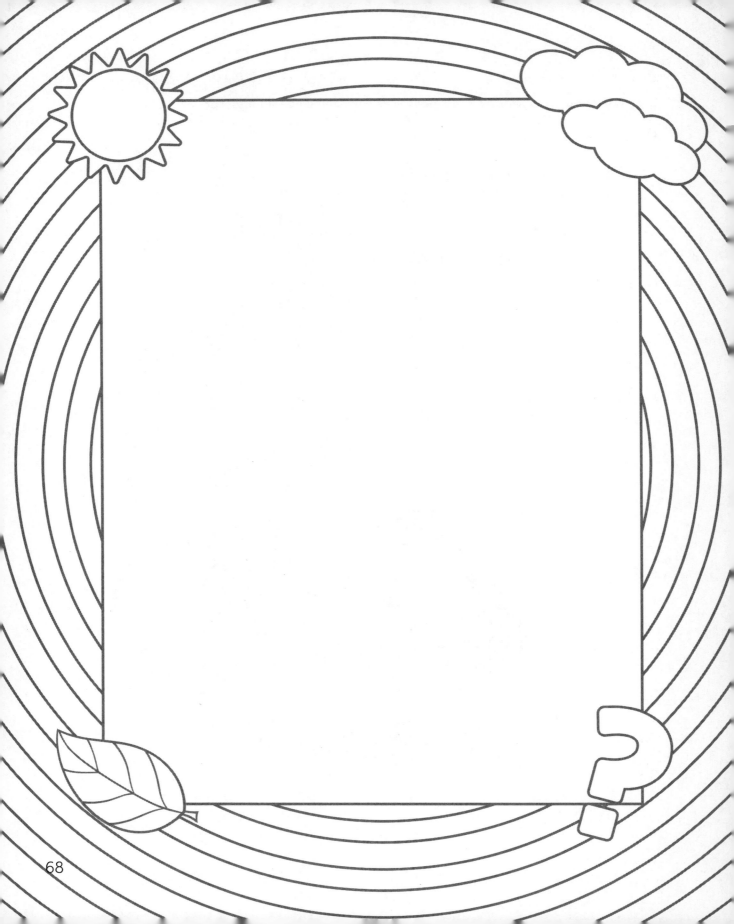

Chapter 6

MASTERING YOUR EMOTIONS

Now that you know how to master your thoughts, let's talk about feelings! The first thing to know is that if you're human, you're going to have all the emotions. If you turned to this chapter hoping for a way to switch off difficult feelings forever, you may be disappointed. You can't get rid of feelings (sorry!). But don't be discouraged. In this chapter, you'll discover why you wouldn't want to, even if you could.

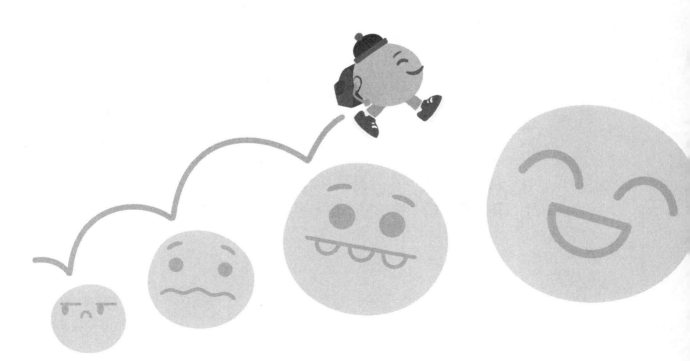

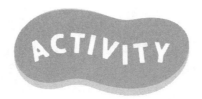

ACTIVITY

EMOTION WORDS

See if you can find the hidden feeling words below. Use a crayon or colored pencil that matches the feeling to circle or highlight each word.

```
D O V E R W H E L M E D A S
R I I N S G D C E M E N E S
A G D E D T I O U A G C Y T
S C E S R N S N L R I A I G
C N T C E A A F Y O I D L E
A D S T H T P I O A A A U S
R S U D J O P D J W G S F U
E T G I B J O E P I I H E R
D E S N O E I N G A T A P P
Y R I S R A N T G F A M O R
O P D D E L T L D D T E H I
F O P D D O E S E E E D S S
N A D A M U D E D C D H D E
I P D O H S D U O R P T U D
```

HAPPY   SAD   ANGRY   SURPRISED   DISAPPOINTED

DISGUSTED   PROUD   BORED   ASHAMED   AGITATED

SCARED   CONFIDENT   OVERWHELMED   JEALOUS   HOPEFUL

HOW DOES IT FEEL?

Emotions are also called *feelings*. They are sensations you feel in your body. They show up in response to things happening around you or thoughts going through your mind. They're like messengers: They visit to give you important information about what's going on. Some are nice to feel, and some are not! Some feel big and intense, and some feel small and gentle. Just like you are not your thoughts, you are also not your feelings. You **have** feelings, and they can sometimes lead to urges to do things. But feelings can't make you do anything; you have choices. For example, when you feel angry, you can choose to take a deep breath and walk away. Or you can choose to throw something across the room! **You** are in control of your actions even when intense emotions show up.

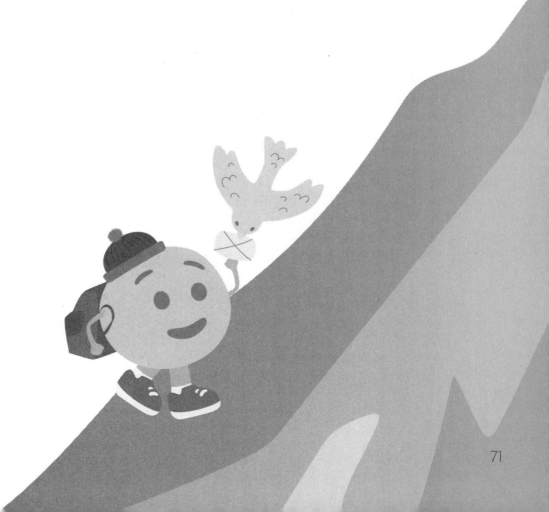

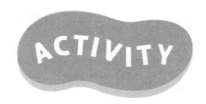

TRY A BODY SCAN

An exercise called a **body scan** can help you notice what you're feeling in your body. It can also remind you that your feelings are just part of what's happening inside and around you. Here's how to do it.

Lie down or sit comfortably; close your eyes, if that feels comfortable. Take a deep breath in, then let it out. Notice the sensations in your body, moving your attention slowly from head to toe. Imagine you have a flashlight and you're shining the light over each part of your body. Stay curious about what you might notice. What feelings, or sensations, can you feel on the outside of your body (like the feeling of your socks or shoes on your feet)? Next, notice the sensations you can feel on the inside of your body (like your heart beating or your lungs filling up with air). Some sensations may be strong and noticeable, and some may be less strong. Notice whether the sensations are comfortable or uncomfortable.

What is it like to be aware of more than one sensation at once?

_____

_____

_____

See if you can let the feelings be there, just as they are, without trying to change them.

Taking the time to notice the sensations in your body gives you clues about your emotions. After the body scan, use colors, shapes, designs, or words inside the clouds on the following page to show what different emotions feel like in your body.

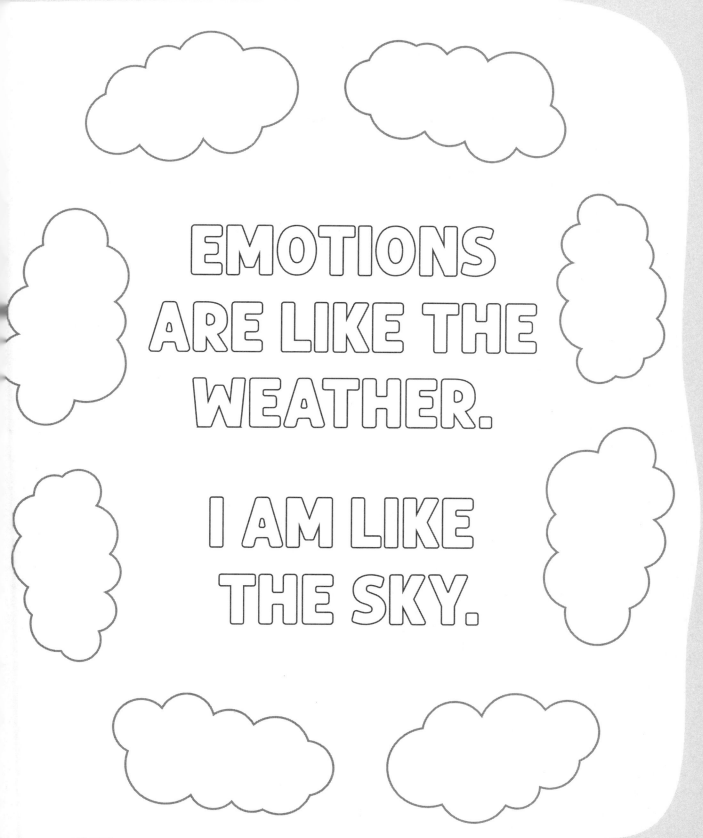

EMOTIONS ARE LIKE THE WEATHER.

I AM LIKE THE SKY.

WHAT'S YOUR WEATHER LIKE?

What's your favorite kind of weather? A hot summer's day? Being cozy inside when it's raining? Everyone likes something different, based on what is more comfortable and enjoyable for them.

What about when it comes to emotions? There are different kinds of feelings, like different kinds of weather. You'll be more comfortable with some emotions than others based on how they feel in your body and what happens when you show them to others. Below, write which emotions you are comfortable having and showing, and which ones you struggle with or don't like to show. **HINT:** You can use the emotion words from the word search on page 70, or come up with your own.

COMFORTABLE FEELINGS	UNCOMFORTABLE FEELINGS

Just like there is no weather that's only "good" or "bad" (we need both sunshine and rain), there are no "good" or "bad" emotions. Emotions are part of being human, and they all have important messages for us. Learning how to **accept** (get okay with) the whole range of emotions will let you keep climbing, no matter the weather. And understanding what our feelings are trying to tell us can help us accept them—even uncomfortable ones.

Below, draw a line from the name of the emotion to the message it tells.

HAPPINESS   I don't feel seen and heard. Do people even like me?

SADNESS   I don't know what's going to happen. I might not be
                   able to handle it.

ANGER   I like this. I am enjoying myself!

ANXIETY   I've lost something important. I miss it a lot.

STRESS   Everything is good right now.

LONELINESS   This is gross and yucky.

DISGUST   This is unfair and wrong! It's **really** not okay with me.

CONTENTMENT   I can't manage this! It's too much.

When a feeling shows up, you can use mindfulness skills (chapter 4). Skills like the body scan help you notice the sensations you feel in your body and be curious about the messages your emotions have for you. Then, you can use self-compassion (chapter 4) to help yourself be more comfortable until the uncomfortable feeling passes.

The next time a difficult emotion is passing through with a message for you, try these steps:

1. What am I feeling? (Notice your feeling, and name it.)

2. Where do I feel it in my body? (Do a body scan to see which sensations are there, and think about which are connected to the emotion.)

3. What is the feeling telling me? (If the feeling could talk, what would it say?)

4. What do I need to be more comfortable while I feel this way? (Would it help to be alone for a while, or to talk to someone you trust, or listen to your favorite song, or...?)

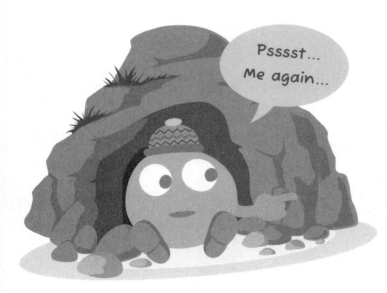

Pssssst... Me again...

If all you feel is empty or numb, that's okay. This can happen when emotions become too intense or go on for too long. Your brain is trying to help you by switching off your ability to notice what you're feeling. You can try noticing other sensations: give yourself a squeezy hug, or feel warmth from a hot chocolate or hot shower, or go outside and feel the sun or breeze on your skin. It's a good idea to let a trusted adult know you're feeling empty or numb. If they know, they can support you.

BONUS ACTIVITY In the back of this book, you'll find an emotional weather chart. You can use this to track how you feel from day to day. It can remind you that all emotions—no matter how strong they are when they show up—are just passing through.

WELCOMING THE WEATHER

It's time for some math! (Yes, you are still in the right workbook...).

Pop quiz:

$3 \times 1 =$

$3 \times 100 =$

$3 \times 10,000 =$

$3 \times 0 =$

$3,000 \times 0 =$

So...why are we doing math when you're here to learn about feelings? Because there's an equation for pain and emotions:

EMOTIONAL PAIN X RESISTANCE = SUFFERING

Let's break it down:

1. Emotional pain = This hurts!
2. Resistance = I'm going to fight it, ignore it, or pretend it's not happening!
3. Suffering = I feel worse, and the pain is going on and on!

This equation tells us that if we have lots of pain but zero resistance, we don't experience suffering (which goes on and on), just the pain (which happens, and then goes away):

3,000 pain x 0 resistance = 0 suffering

It also tells us that if we have just a little bit of pain but **lots** of resistance, we're going to suffer a lot on top of the pain we started with.

3 pain x 1,000 resistance = 3,000 suffering

It turns out people are pretty good at dealing with pain when we have to. We're **not** so good at handling suffering. What's the difference? Life can serve up all kinds of painful moments we can't avoid:

- Rock in your shoe   **= PAIN**

- Blister from your hiking boot   **= PAIN**

- A pet dying   **= PAIN**

- Parents getting a divorce   **= PAIN**

- Moving far away from your best friend   **= PAIN**

All these things truly hurt—**and** people have survived painful situations and emotions since time began. Since painful things happen, our brains and bodies are built to help us handle them.

Now check out these examples of suffering:

- Pretending you're fine because you believe people will think you're weak for being upset about your pet dying   **= SUFFERING**

- Blaming yourself for your parents' divorce   **= SUFFERING**

- Avoiding kids in your new town because you're scared to make new friends in case you move again   **= SUFFERING**

- Bottling up your emotions because you don't want to worry your parents   **= SUFFERING**

The bottom line? We can't avoid all the painful things in life, but we can reduce how much we suffer. Again, resistance turns pain (which happens sometimes to everyone) into suffering (which is often unnecessary).

Remember the saying earlier in the workbook, "Name it to tame it, feel it to heal it"? It means if we notice and name what's hurting us, and feel the real pain from that hurt, the hurt can start to heal. **Resistance** is when we do the opposite. Resistance means ignoring your feelings (or pushing them down or bottling them up); avoiding dealing with things that are happening; blaming yourself for things going wrong; or doing any of the behaviors on the avoidance list (page 24) to try and get rid of your pain or hide it from others. The more you resist dealing with your actual pain, the more you suffer.

Think of it like this. Imagine having a rock in your shoe while you're mountain climbing—**painful**! If you ignore it because you don't want to look slow or weak, that's **resistance.** You're going to **suffer** a lot more and have a much bigger injury. If you **accept** that you have a rock in your shoe (and that you'll be in pain until it's out) and pause to deal with it, what's likely to happen?

It might cost you a few minutes on the climb. You might have some pain from where the rock poked your foot. But you're going to **suffer** a lot less—both while you're hiking and afterward, when your foot is healing.

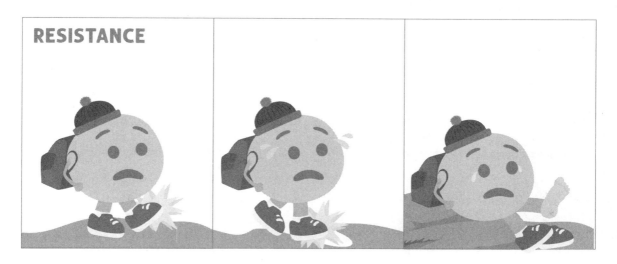

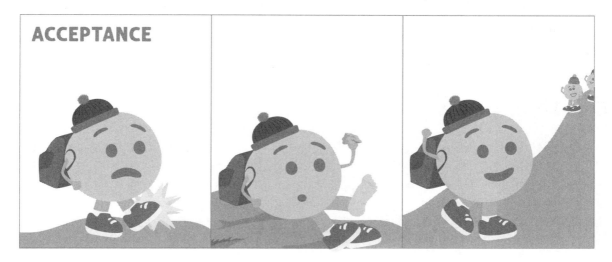

Draw a picture of (or describe) a painful situation you've experienced. Include what emotions you felt:

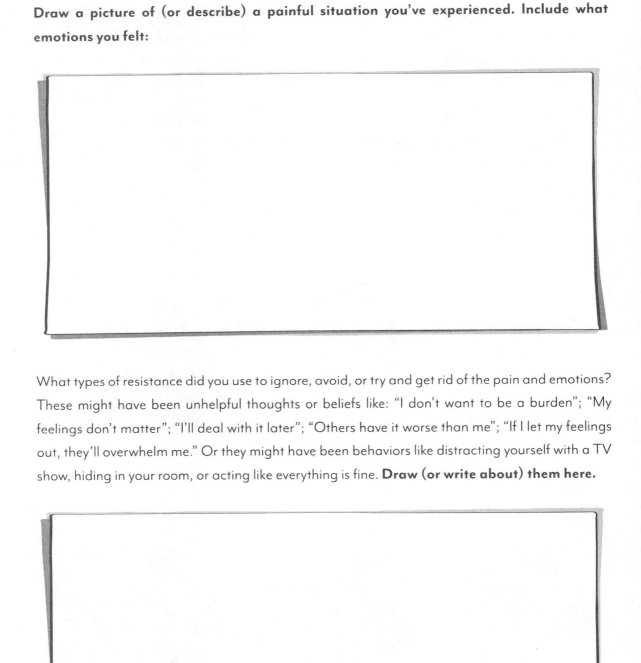

What types of resistance did you use to ignore, avoid, or try and get rid of the pain and emotions? These might have been unhelpful thoughts or beliefs like: "I don't want to be a burden"; "My feelings don't matter"; "I'll deal with it later"; "Others have it worse than me"; "If I let my feelings out, they'll overwhelm me." Or they might have been behaviors like distracting yourself with a TV show, hiding in your room, or acting like everything is fine. **Draw (or write about) them here.**

What extra suffering did you have because of the resistance? For example: "The problem lasted longer or got worse"; "I felt worse about myself"; "No one knew I was in pain so no one helped me"). **Draw (or write about) it here.**

What might have happened if you accepted the painful situation and its emotions, and showed yourself compassion? Would you have suffered less, even if the situation didn't change? **Draw (or write about) a different ending here:**

If you've grown up being told ideas like:

- Your feelings don't matter

- You're a burden

- You're too sensitive

- Having (or showing) emotions is weak

or any other unhelpful or unkind idea, I'm truly sorry. You've been given bad information. Those things simply are not true. You may not believe it yet, but the truth about life, emotions, and everything (okay, maybe not quite everything) is on the next page...

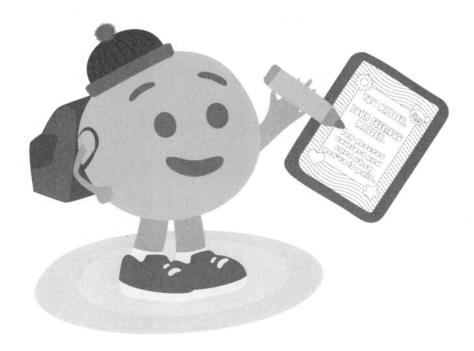

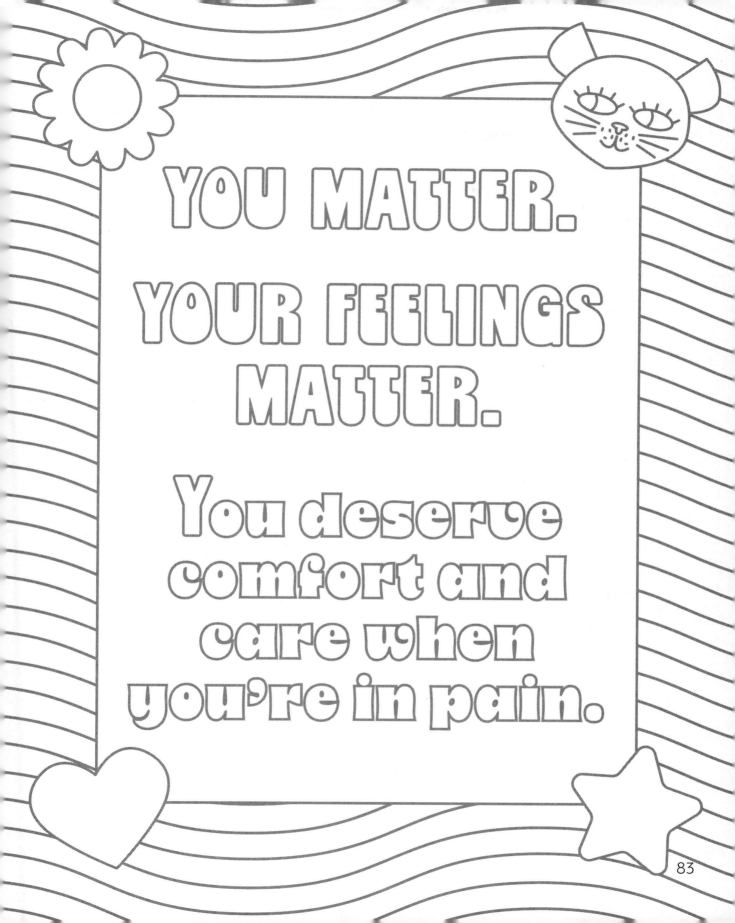

YOU MATTER.
YOUR FEELINGS MATTER.

You deserve comfort and care when you're in pain.

83

A CARE PACKAGE JUST FOR YOU

Imagine the sun is setting on the mountain and you're settling in for the night. The temperature is dropping, the wind is picking up, and the clouds are dark and heavy. You're in for a rainy, cold, windy night. List or draw pictures of some items you would like to receive in a care package. **What would help you be more comfortable on this cold, stormy night on the mountain?**

These things won't fix the bad weather. But they can make your night on the mountain better.

Sometimes there's nothing you can do to change a painful situation or the strong emotions that visit with it. The best way to help yourself through it is to comfort yourself, the way you would comfort a friend or a loved one. **Draw (or write about) something that would feel comforting (and safe) for each of these:**

Something to comfort my body (like: a fluffy blanket, petting a cat, warm bath)

Something to comfort my mind (like: playing a favorite song, looking at cute or funny animal videos)

Something to help me feel safe (like: being around friends or family, talking to someone about the problem, getting rid of hurtful things)

IMPORTANT: Some of the ways you comfort yourself may look like the avoidance behaviors on page 24. This is confusing, right? The difference is **why** you're doing the behavior. If you're doing it to try and get rid of your pain or emotions, that's avoidance (or resistance), and it won't help you in the long run. If you're doing it to make yourself more comfortable while the pain or emotion is visiting, that's acceptance, and it can help.

This chapter started with disappointing news—that you can't get rid of uncomfortable feelings. Now you know it's normal for people to experience the whole range of emotions, and feelings bring important messages. You can suffer less by accepting the painful things in life, welcoming all your feelings when they visit, and comforting yourself when things are tough.

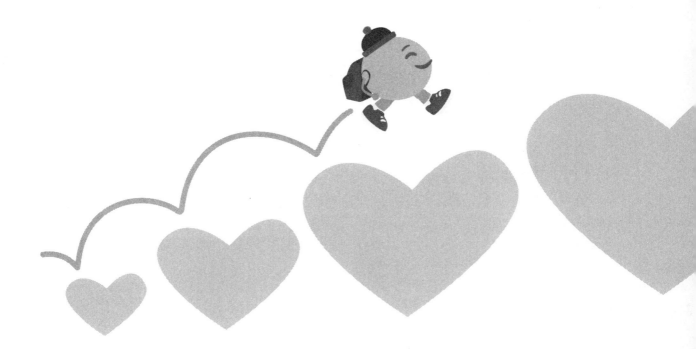

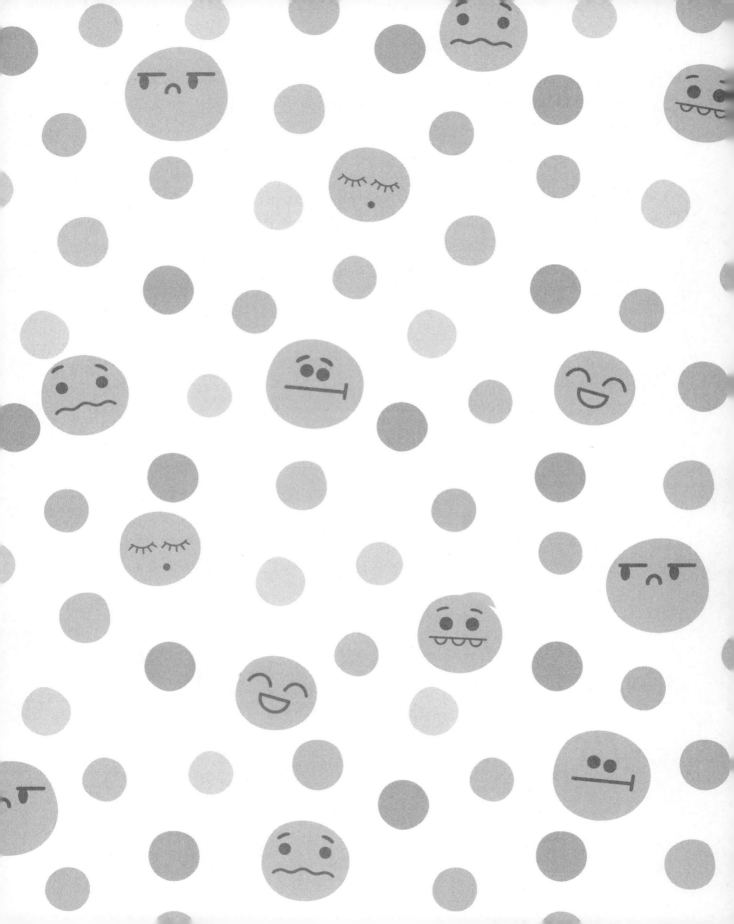

Chapter 7

MASTERING RELATIONSHIPS

Here's something true about all humans: People need other people to survive! It's just how we are. Being connected to other people helps us grow and makes life meaningful.

Up until now, your main relationships have probably been with your family. As you keep climbing the mountain toward your teenage years and into adulthood, friends are a more important part of your life. Who you surround yourself with can matter a lot to your mental health, and to how you feel about yourself as a person.

Because relationships are so important (and can be tricky), this chapter will add relationship skills to your pack.

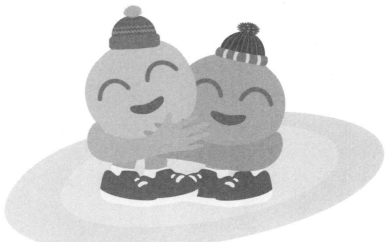

A REASON, A SEASON, OR A LIFETIME

It's been said there are three main types of relationships—people you meet for a reason, for a season, or for a lifetime. These climbing companions share your journey for a while or for the long haul.

People who come into your life for a reason are those who teach you something, meet a need, or help you discover something about yourself. Think of someone who teaches you how to pitch your tent on your first night mountain climbing but takes a different path the next morning. Without them you would have really struggled, and you might feel disappointed you didn't get more time together. But their job is done, and you might not see them again.

Some people travel with you for a while—a "season" of time. The season might be short or long. You might go through a lot together. They might help you grow as a person or reach a goal. Then the season ends, and your relationship changes or fades away. Think of it as meeting someone who is climbing the same route on the mountain as you. You buddy up for part of the journey. You might overcome obstacles together, share stories, make memories, and help each other along the way. At some point your paths take you in different directions and it's time to say goodbye. You'll miss their company, and you'll look back fondly on the time you shared.

A few special people will join you for the lifetime journey. No matter what happens or how far apart you live, they'll always be there. When you see each other again it will feel like no time has passed. They'll see you at your best and your worst. They'll accept you just as you are. Think of meeting someone on the mountain who just gets you! They truly like you for you. Even if you go off on different tracks, when you meet up, you're excited to see them. You encourage each other to keep going. You can always turn to them for love and support.

As you make your own way up the mountain, you'll meet lots of different people. all with a role to play in your life. You'll have a role to play in theirs too. It can be difficult when relationships change or end, but you now have skills that will help. You can use acceptance when relationships end or change. You can practice self-compassion for any pain you feel.

Think about the people you have known.

Who was someone who was in your life for a reason**? What did they teach you or help you with?**

_____

_____

_____

_____

Who was someone who was in your life for a season**? What season did you share together? How did it feel when the relationship changed?**

_____

_____

_____

_____

Who is someone you hope will be in your life forever? What about them makes them a special person to have on the journey?

_____

_____

_____

_____

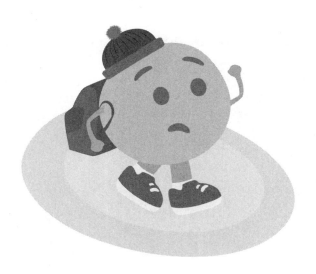

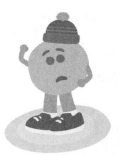

Relationships ending or changing can be sad or hard. **What is something kind and supportive you can say to yourself when a relationship changes or comes to an end?**

_____

_____

_____

_____

_____

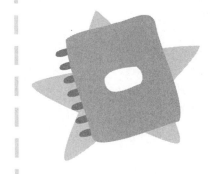

BONUS ACTIVITY Photo journals are a great way to store memories. In a journal (online or in a paper notebook), add photos of the people in your life and your adventures together. As you get older, you can look back and remember special people who came into your life, moments you shared, and lessons they taught you.

FINDING THE RIGHT CLIMBING CREW

The people you spend time with have a big influence on your life, so choose your crew wisely! Figuring out friendships can feel like cracking a code that other people already know. It can be hard to know who to trust, what to share about yourself, and what to accept in each friendship.

Unscramble the words below to uncover qualities of healthy friendships.

RICANG

WRUTHTROSTY

UNF

PESTFULREC

THONES

PURTIVESOP

RISTEDENT

What other qualities do you try to show as a good friend?

How does it feel when you're with people who accept you just as you are?

A NOTE ON BULLYING

Fun fact—no one your age is a friendship expert! Everyone is new to it and is figuring it out as they go. Sometimes people are struggling more than we know. When people are under stress it can change their behavior. They may do and say things that aren't kind.

If someone is being unkind to you (in person or online), it can be tricky to know how to handle it. A good response is one that

- gets the other person to think about their behavior,

- communicates that you don't like how they are acting, and

- doesn't involve you also acting in unkind ways.

Here are some phrases to use if someone is being unkind to you. Circle or highlight the ones you might use.

- That was an unkind thing to say/do. Are you okay?

- Did you mean to say that out loud?

- We all say things we'll regret. Do you need a minute?

- It seems like you're struggling. I'm going to give you some space.

- I don't like being talked to that way. I'm done with this conversation.

These kinds of responses may take the other person by surprise (it's probably not the reaction they were expecting). More importantly, they help communicate that you're not going to react with your own unkind thoughts, words, or actions. When people see they aren't going to get a reaction out of you, they usually back off.

As best you can, don't let others' unkind words or opinions stick in your mind. If someone handed you a sticky note that said "you're the worst person ever," you **could** choose to stick it on your chest and walk around believing it forever. Or you could scrunch it up and throw it away. You don't need to hold on to unkind words!

If your brain gets stuck repeating or replaying unkind thoughts:

- Check those thoughts: are they true/helpful/kind?

- Revisit ways to separate from your thoughts (page 65).

- Give yourself compassion for any uncomfortable feelings that visit with the thoughts.

If you're the target of persistent unkindness from others, that's bullying. It's important that you let a trusted adult know so they can support you. If you need to, use the help request card at the back of this book to let an adult know what's going on!

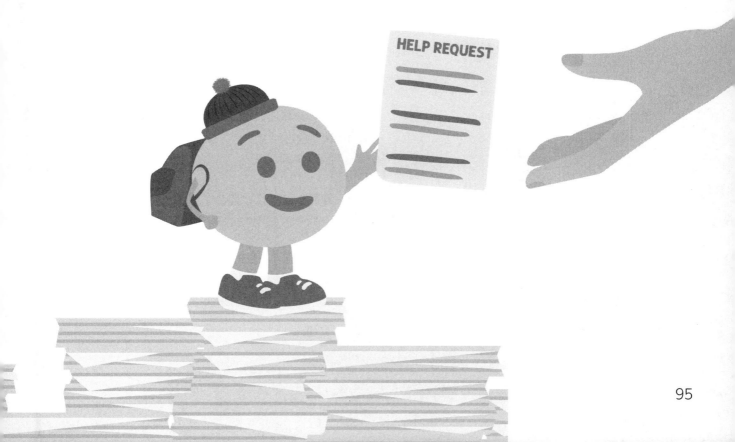

WHAT ABOUT FITTING IN?

Right now, a lot of voices may be telling you what to do, who you should be, and what matters most. It can be tempting to follow the crowd and try to fit in. No one wants to feel left out or left behind. That would be scary! In fact, feeling like you belong to a group is one of the most important things to preteen and teen brains. Feeling different and alone hurts.

The truth is, some of the things you like and that matter to you may also matter to the people around you. Some won't. As a preteen, you're starting to have more of your own ideas. You'll want to express yourself in your own way and decide for yourself what you care about. (We'll talk about your values and goals in the next chapter.) It can be tricky when you and your friends start liking different things.

So how do you balance wanting to belong and wanting to be yourself? Boundary skills and communication skills can really help.

BOUNDARIES help do two things—keep things out and keep things in. Imagine a sign on the mountain that says, "Trail closed due to falling rocks." The sign keeps climbers safe from falling rocks. It sets a boundary that helps keep you safe. Setting healthy boundaries helps you stay safe and protect what is important to you.

Trail closed due to falling rocks.

Here are some examples of healthy boundaries:

- building trust slowly in relationships
- telling people how you feel and what you need
- asking someone to stop, if what they are doing or saying is hurting or upsetting you
- having control over what happens to your body
- requesting privacy or space
- having your own belief system
- deciding what is important to you
- using "No" as a full sentence (you don't always have to explain it)

Can you think of boundaries that are important to you? Write them here:

TALKING ABOUT BOUNDARIES

Sometimes we need to let other people know about our boundaries. This can be tricky! We might worry about how the other person will react or what they'll think about us.

Do you have any fears about communicating your boundaries to other people?

_____

_____

_____

_____

_____

How we communicate our boundaries influences how other people hear and respond to us. There are three main ways people communicate: **passive**, **assertive**, and **aggressive**.

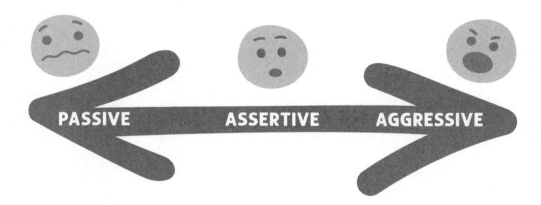

Passive communication is when you try to communicate something without actually saying it. Think of turning your head away when someone takes the last donut (that you wanted). **Assertive communication** is when you say what you mean without being rude or unkind: "Hey, could we split that donut? I haven't had one yet." **Aggressive communication** is like an attack. It can be loud, and even scary to the other person: "Get your hand off that donut! It's mine!"

Since it's honest and doesn't attack the other person, assertive communication is the best way to communicate boundaries. Being clear, calm, and confident shows you respect yourself and the other person. When you passively communicate your boundaries, the other person probably won't understand what you're trying to say. When you're aggressive, the other person could feel like you're attacking them.

With assertive communication, you can say what you need from another person. This shows them they can do the same thing. A conversation where each person can say what they want or need and can listen to and respect the other person is a conversation with good boundaries!

Here's a script to help use assertive communication and let someone know what your boundaries are.

> **I feel** [say how you feel] **when you** [describe what they're doing]. **What I would like is** [say what you'd like instead—your boundary]. **Otherwise** [say how you'll respond if they cross your boundary].

For example: **I felt** hurt and betrayed **when you** told everyone I believe in the abominable snowman. **What I would like is** for you to keep it between us when I share personal things with you. **Otherwise**, I'll stop sharing personal things with you, which will change our friendship.

Below are some situations where a preteen needs to communicate a boundary. See if you can identify which communication style they're using (passive, assertive, or aggressive). Then help them find an assertive way of getting their message across.

SITUATION 1 Chloe's friend keeps messaging late at night asking for advice on a problem they're having. Chloe wants to be a good friend, but she's getting in trouble with her parents for being on her phone. She's also struggling to concentrate at school after the late nights. Chloe wants to tell her friend she can't keep messaging after she's gone to bed. The next day she tells her friend she's really tired. But that night she still texts them back even though it's super late.

Is this a **PASSIVE / ASSERTIVE / AGGRESSIVE** way to communicate a boundary? (**circle one**)

Help Chloe assertively let her friend know what her boundary is by filling in the gaps below:

I feel _____ when you _____ .

What I would like is _____ . Otherwise _____ .

SITUATION 2 Noah likes playing soccer at recess. Every day as they head out to the field, Noah's friends make jokes about how he's out of shape and slow. Noah used to laugh it off but it's really starting to bother him. Today he's decided he's had enough, and he tells his friends where they can shove their soccer ball, then he kicks it over the fence and storms off.

Is this a **PASSIVE / ASSERTIVE / AGGRESSIVE** way to communicate a boundary? (circle one)

Help Noah assertively let his friends know what his boundary is by filling in the gaps below:

I feel _____ when you _____ .

What I would like is _____ . Otherwise _____ .

SITUATION 3 Padma is going to a family dinner and her grandparents will be there. She's always been taught that it's polite to give them a hug and kiss to say hello and goodbye, but she just doesn't feel comfortable doing that anymore. She begs her parents not to make her go, but doesn't tell them why. They get frustrated and tell Padma she's being "moody."

Is this a **PASSIVE / ASSERTIVE / AGGRESSIVE** way to communicate a boundary? (**circle one**)

Help Padma assertively let her parents know what her boundary is by filling in the gaps below:

I feel _____ when Grandma and Grandpa _____ .

What I would like is _____ . Otherwise _____ .

Now think of a boundary that's important to you. Write down what it is, and how you could assertively communicate it.

My boundary: _____

How I can assertively communicate my boundary to _____ [insert someone's name]:

_____

 If this skill is important for you, add "assertively communicating my boundaries" to your skill tracker.

PARENTS ARE PEOPLE, TOO

As you journey through your preteen years, your relationships will start to change. Friends become more important, and your relationship with the adults raising you (AKA your parents/caregivers) changes. The adults are expecting this but that doesn't mean they know how to handle it. Up until now, they've been like the tour guides on your mountain climbing adventure. They've led the way, made the plans, fixed the problems, and told you what to do. As you're growing up and wanting to go on adventures on your own and with friends, the adults become more like climbing coaches. They're there to give you tips, ideas, and encouragement, but they won't necessarily go on every adventure with you. This transition can be tough, and every family handles it differently.

Here are four things parents/caregivers of preteens wish their young people knew. (Brace yourself, it's going to be a little bit mushy.)

- They love you more than you could possibly imagine. Even when they're mad. Even when they don't know how to show it. Even when you mess up.

- They hurt when you hurt, which is why they sometimes try to "fix" things, rather than just listening when you vent.

- You're not a burden, and it won't "worry them more" if you tell them what's going on.

- They're slightly terrified of you climbing up the mountain without them by your side. But they're also so excited for you to go and have your own adventures.

What's something you appreciate about what the adults in your life have taught you, done for you, or prepared you for?

_____

_____

_____

_____

What are some things you wish the adults raising you knew about you and what it's like being a preteen?

_____

_____

_____

_____

BONUS ACTIVITY If you're feeling brave, you could share this page with the important adults in your life. They might have other things they want to share with you. And they would love to know the things you wish they knew.

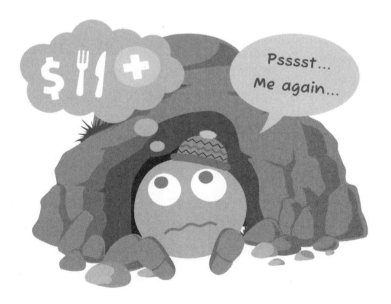

Not all parents/caregivers have the skills or resources they need to take good care of their kids. If the adults in your home are struggling to take care of you or keep you safe, please use the help request card in the back of this book. Give it to a trusted adult (a relative or neighbor, or someone at your school, sports club, place of worship, or doctor's office) so they can help you.

DON'T FORGET ME...

There is another very important relationship in your life. It started the day you were born: It's the relationship you have with yourself. **If you haven't met yourself yet, take a moment to say "hello" and introduce yourself. (You can use the prompts below.)**

Self Portrait

Write down five unique qualities about yourself:

Write a list of (or draw) your favorite things:

Write about (or draw pictures of) your perfect day:

Your relationship with yourself is the ultimate lifelong friendship. There's no one else on the planet who knows just what it's like to be you. That means you can decide: Are you going to be a good friend to yourself or are you going to be a bully?

What would it look like if you treated yourself like you were your own best friend?

Pick one (or more) of the best-friend promises below and add it to your skill tracker to remind you of your promise to yourself.

- I will speak to myself with kindness.
- I will take the best possible care of myself I can.
- I will take time to get to know myself well.
- I will encourage myself when things are tough.
- I will spend time doing things I enjoy.
- I will be honest with myself.
- _____

BONUS ACTIVITY How excited would you be if you got to see your best friend every single morning? For the next week, try looking in the mirror and saying, "Good morning, friend." Then remind yourself of the promise you chose above. You could give yourself a high-five, a smile, or some words of encouragement to start your day and remind yourself to be your own best friend.

Now that you have the skills to master the important relationships in your life, it's time to journey into the future!

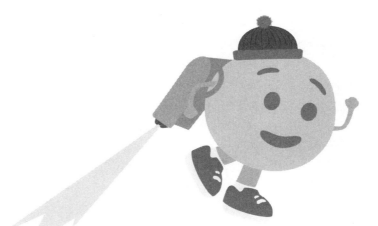

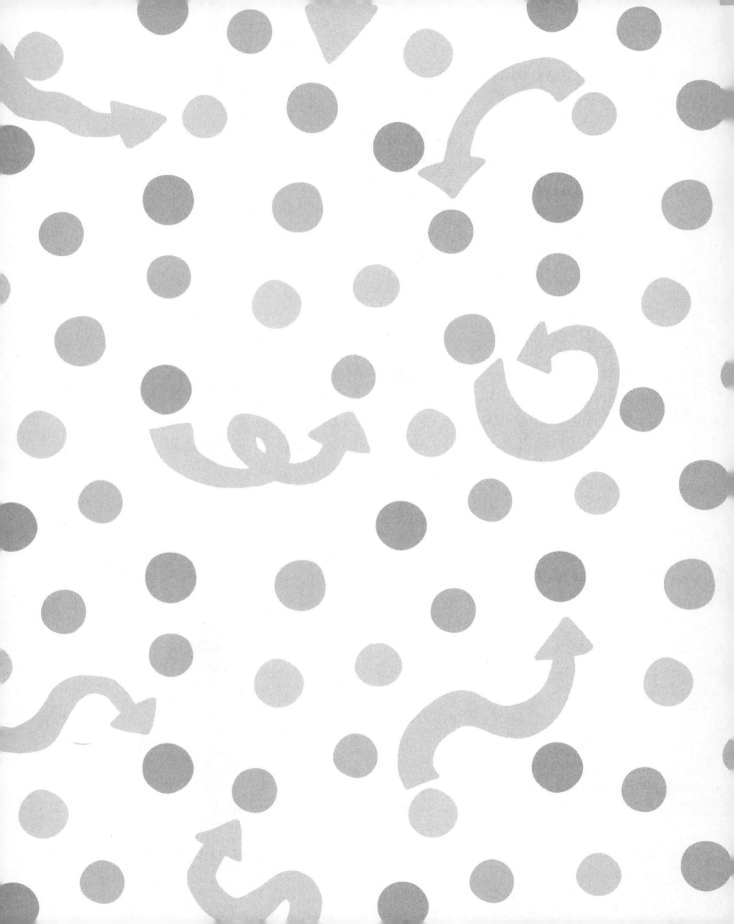

Chapter 8

MASTERING YOUR FUTURE

There's a saying: "It's not where you start but where you end up that matters." Things may be tough right now, but you won't be a preteen forever. Things will change. Now that your pack is loaded with useful skills for your journey though the preteen years, it's time to set off on your climb. While no one knows exactly what the future holds, you get to **choose** the direction you want for your life. Making a mindful choice about who you want to be and what's important in life will help you reach your goals and notice when things are getting off track.

This chapter will help you figure out what's most important to you so you can keep moving toward the life you want!

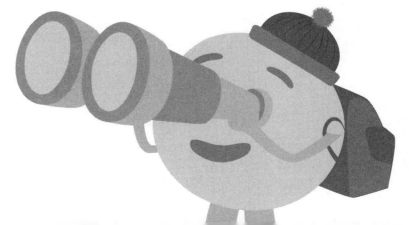

UNCOVER WHAT MATTERS TO YOU

What matters most to you? What kind of person do you want to be? Answering these questions can help you name your **values**. They are like a compass (or a GPS) keeping you on track.

Answering these questions can help you discover some of your values.

What helpful lessons or ideas have my family tried to teach me?

_____

_____

_____

_____

What personal qualities do the people I admire have?

_____

_____

_____

_____

What qualities do I hope people see in me through how I act and treat others?

_____

_____

_____

_____

If I could achieve anything in life, what would it be?

_____

_____

_____

_____

_____

Looking at your answers, use the list of values below and highlight the five things that matter most to you right now.

Acceptance	Determination	Learning
Achievement	Diversity	Mastery
Balance	Enjoyment	Openness
Belonging	Excellence	Persistence
Bravery	Fairness	Resilience
Caring	Flexibility	Resourcefulness
Contentment	Freedom	Respect
Courage	Generosity	Simplicity
Contribution	Growth	Solitude
Creativity	Health	Security
Curiosity	Honesty	Teamwork
Dependability	Independence	Trust

Use the next page to create a poster of your top five values. Include words and pictures showing the things that matter most to you.

How can your values help you make decisions about your future? Great question! **Think about a problem you're facing right now, that you're not sure how to get through. Write it below:**

_____

_____

_____

Now look at your top five values. What would a person who has those qualities and beliefs do? For example, if you value determination, what would a determined person do in this situation? If you value honesty, what would an honest person do? **Based on** your **values, what steps could you take to help yourself with the problem?**

_____

_____

_____

_____

_____

_____

When you make decisions based on your values (not just thoughts or emotions), you're more likely to keep moving toward what matters most to you. For example, if you really value honesty, but you're nervous about telling the truth about something, it can be hard to decide what to do. Take some time to think about it. What would happen if you were led by the uncomfortable feeling or the worrying thoughts? How likely are you to tell the truth? What would happen if you used your values to decide what to do? If you're ever unsure about what to do, look at your top five values poster to help you make a wise and kind decision.

SETTING GOALS

Now that you know what's most important to you, you can set some goals. **Goals** are things you want to work toward or achieve. They can be big or small, and once you reach them, you can set a new goal to help you keep moving forward. If you have a bigger goal, try breaking it down into smaller steps.

Let's set a goal based on one of your top five values.

The value I choose is

The goal I have is

How long do I think it will take to reach this goal?

I'll know I've reached my goal when

The tools from my pack that can help me reach my goal are

Other tools, information, or support I might need to reach my goal are

The first three small steps I can take toward this goal are:

1.

2.

3.

HINT: If you like, add a reminder of this goal to your vision board.

FAILURE, SUCCESS, AND PERFECTION

Lots of preteens are hard on themselves—especially when their goals or plans don't work out. It's normal to feel disappointed. Some people (including adults) find disappointment so uncomfortable that they'll do anything to avoid it. They may decide that if they never try, they can't fail. Or they may go overboard to make sure they won't fail (like staying up all night to study for a test).

Some people believe they've already failed or are a failure. They think there's no point trying new or difficult things. Have you ever had thoughts like these? **Put a check next to any that sound familiar:**

- ☐ There's no point trying; I can't do it anyway.
- ☐ If I don't get good grades, people will think I'm stupid.
- ☐ Winning is the only thing that matters.
- ☐ If you expect the worst, you can't get hurt.
- ☐ People will only like me if I do well.
- ☐ Doing well now means I must do even better next time.
- ☐ If it's not perfect, it's ruined.
- ☐ Failure is not an option.
- ☐ _____

These are all unhelpful ideas. If you checked any, where did those come from? They may have come from a family member or other important person in your life. (Hold that thought: You can use it in the cloudy vision exercise later in this chapter.) Or they may have shown up in your mind all by themselves.

Wherever they came from, unhelpful beliefs won't help you get to the summit. Why? Because failure is an important part of learning. No one masters something on their first try. Everyone has to start at the beginning and learn through making mistakes, trying again, and figuring things out.

People who achieve great things often celebrate when they get things wrong. They know failure means they're one step closer to achieving their goal. Their motto is: "To fail is to succeed at trying." You need to be willing to get things wrong and do things imperfectly if you want to get better at something. Perfection doesn't exist in the real world. But success does. And whether you've succeeded or not is based on your values—what is most important to you. Since everyone's values are unique, success is different for everyone.

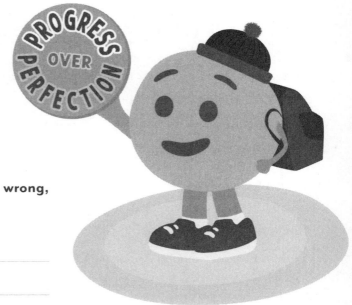

Write something you've failed at, gotten wrong, or messed up:

_____

_____

_____

_____

_____

What did you learn from things not working out? Did this mistake mean:

    a) You're a failure, and should never try anything ever again in life.

    or

    b) You're still learning, and everyone makes mistakes.

HINT: If you chose (a), please run that thought through the true/helpful/kind filter, then try again.

It comes down to this: Are you willing to make mistakes in life to get better at the things that matter most to you?

Below, write a helpful reminder that you can look back on next time you make a mistake, or things don't go as you planned. (Find some quotes about failure and success to inspire you!)

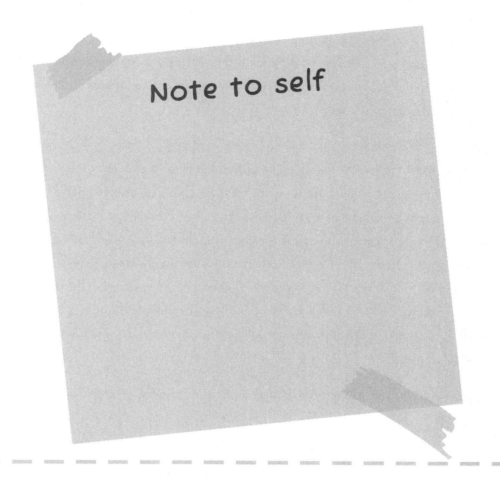

Note to self

BONUS TIP People who are more compassionate toward themselves tend to achieve higher in school and reach more of their goals. That's because people who know how to:

- notice their thoughts and feelings,

- comfort themselves, and

- remind themselves everyone makes mistakes

are better at picking themselves up and trying again, instead of beating themselves up and deciding to quit!

CLEAR VISION AND CLOUDY VISION

Some days on the mountain of life are going to be clear and crisp, and it will be easy to see where you're going. Other days—particularly when you're going through the adolescent avalanche—are rainy, misty, even stormy. At times, it may feel like you've forgotten who you are and where you're going. You might get taken off course by the ideas and values of people around you. Or you may feel like you need to hide or change what's important to you to fit in or stay safe. Just like getting swept up in a snowstorm and losing your way, this can be scary.

Take a minute and think about people who influence your life right now. This could be people you know in real life (teachers, friends, relatives, neighbors) or who you follow or talk to online. Use the circles of influence exercise to think about what messages, values, or ideas these people bring to your life. These might be helpful or harmful messages. They could be about how you should live, how you should look, what you should buy, what you should eat, how you should spend your time, and what is important in life. Some online content can give you the message that you're awesome just the way you are—positive, helpful messages. Or content might give you the message that you need to change things about yourself, do certain things, or buy certain things to be okay. These messages aren't actually about you, or what will help you live your life well. This makes them **not** helpful, and possibly hurtful.

Think of your life as a circle inside other circles. The inside circle is your self, including your mind and body and feelings and dreams and talents—everything that makes you, you. The next circle is the people closest to you, who have a big impact on your life. The other circles are people or voices that are farther away from you but still influence how you think and feel. In the outer circle are people you may know of (like celebrities), but who don't know you.

Write the names of people who belong in each circle of your life. Then, outside the circle, write some of the messages you get from these people and voices. Write the ones that help you be your true self on the left. Write the ones that don't support you being exactly who you are on the right. Where are the helpful messages coming from? Where are the messages that suggest you're not okay coming from?

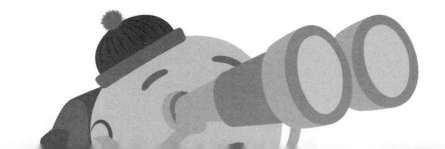

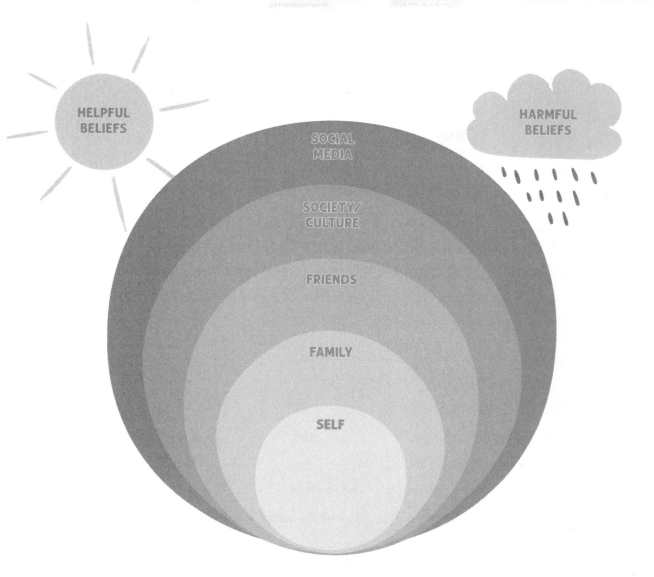

It's absolutely okay to listen to wise and trusted voices in your life—they can offer you guidance, reassurance, or advice about your current situation or your future. If you found some unhelpful messages coming from people and voices in the exercise above, what could you do to minimize the impact these have on your life? Maybe setting and communicating your boundaries could help you stay true to who you are and what's important to you. If you're not sure, that's okay—this is something you can keep paying attention to as you go. And there are ideas in the next section that might help!

BONUS TIP If lots of the unhelpful messages are coming from voices online, it might be time for a social media reset. Go through the list of sites and people you follow and ask yourself if they are helpful or harmful influences on your life. Keep the helpful, unfollow the harmful.

CONTROLLING WHAT YOU CAN

So far, this workbook has focused on things **you can do** to help you through the challenges you're facing as a preteen, survive the adolescent avalanche, and have excellent mental health in adulthood. But what about situations **outside** of your control? Sometimes you can get stuck worrying about things you can't change. This can harm your mood and make it harder to focus on the things within your control.

You might be starting to worry about what will happen during the adolescent avalanche, and what will change when you're a teenager. You might worry about some bigger issues in the world, like climate change. Or maybe there's a situation in your life you can't change right now but that you spend a lot of time thinking or worrying about.

When you spend a lot of time worrying about things outside of your control, it can cause other problems, like those listed below. **Put a check next to any you have experienced.**

- ☐ Difficulty falling asleep
- ☐ Difficulty concentrating
- ☐ Feeling worried or anxious
- ☐ Feeling irritable or annoyed over small things
- ☐ Wanting more control over things like what you eat, what you wear, or where you go
- ☐ Falling behind on schoolwork or daily tasks
- ☐ Struggling to make decisions
- ☐ Saying "no" to things that matter, like going out, doing chores, or spending time with others
- ☐ Getting headaches or feeling sick in your stomach
- ☐ Spending a lot of time zoning out online or with other distractions

Worrying about things outside your control will not help you solve them. And the worrying can cause other areas of your life, like self-care, school, or friendships, to get off course too. You're more likely to stay on track by focusing on the things you can control. Figuring out what those things are is an important skill that will help you for your whole life. **Below, write down any situations or worries you have that are outside of your control.**

FOR LATER

Now, write a list of things **only you** can control right now—for example, going to bed on time, doing your homework, or brushing your teeth. Sometimes you may not be able to solve a big problem (like climate change). But there are small things you can do like saving water and recycling. **Write down as many big and small things you can think of that** you can choose to do **that will help improve your life and your world.**

FOR NOW

Put a check next to things you listed that you're managing well. Circle the ones that need more of your time and attention.

When you notice yourself worrying about things outside of your control, try telling yourself something like:

It's frustrating that I can't solve this right now. I am going to focus on the things I can control and keep my life on track until things change or get clearer.

KEEPING PROBLEMS IN PERSPECTIVE

You've overcome a lot of challenges in your life so far, some big and some small. During the preteen years, as your brain is busy preparing for adolescence, your perspective about things can shift. Small things can start to feel big, and big things can feel enormous. You might notice that your emotions start to become more intense. You might even be surprised by the size of your reaction to things that didn't really bother you before. This has to do with how quickly your brain and body are growing, and it's completely normal. To help keep perspective, you can use a mental scale. (This can also help the people around you who are noticing your emotions have become more intense.)

To start, think about the absolute worst thing you could imagine happening in your life. Write it below. For example: "My house burns down and I lose everything."

Now write down a small inconvenience you've dealt with this past week. For example: "I had to wear my least favorite pair of socks because the others were all dirty."

Your absolute worst thing ("house fire") is a 10 on the scale below, and the small inconvenience ("bad socks") is a 1.

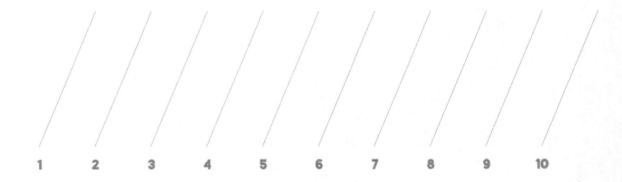

1   2   3   4   5   6   7   8   9   10

Now come up with situations that fall in the middle of the scale. Think about whether each is a bump in the road (1–4)*, a roadblock (5–7)**, or an avalanche (8–10)***. Add these situations to the scale.

* A BUMP IN THE ROAD is something that's a little annoying. It's something you can solve by yourself and move past quickly.

** A ROADBLOCK is going to slow you down for longer. You may need help to clear it from the road, or you may need to find a way around it.

*** AN AVALANCHE is a serious problem. There may be long-term consequences, and you'll definitely need the help of trusted adults to get through it.

Next time you're noticing intense emotions about a challenging situation, come back to this scale and see where the situation fits on the scale. Reminding yourself of the size of the problem can help you keep things in perspective. It can also help you decide whether you can handle the problem on your own or need help.

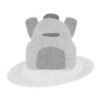
Add "keeping problems in perspective" to your skill tracker, to remind you to come back and use this helpful tool! Knowing the size of a problem can help you figure out what strategies might support you. For example, taking a deep breath will help your body feel calmer while you navigate a bump in the road. But it might not feel like it helps much during an avalanche!

Fortunately, you now have a pack full of useful skills to help you make it to the summit! At the back of the book, you'll find a list of all the skills you've learned. Turn to the list and:

- draw a triangle next to the skills you think would help you with a bump in the road

- draw a square next to the skills that will help you get through a roadblock

- draw a circle next to the skills you need during an avalanche

HINT: Some skills can help with more than one size of problem.

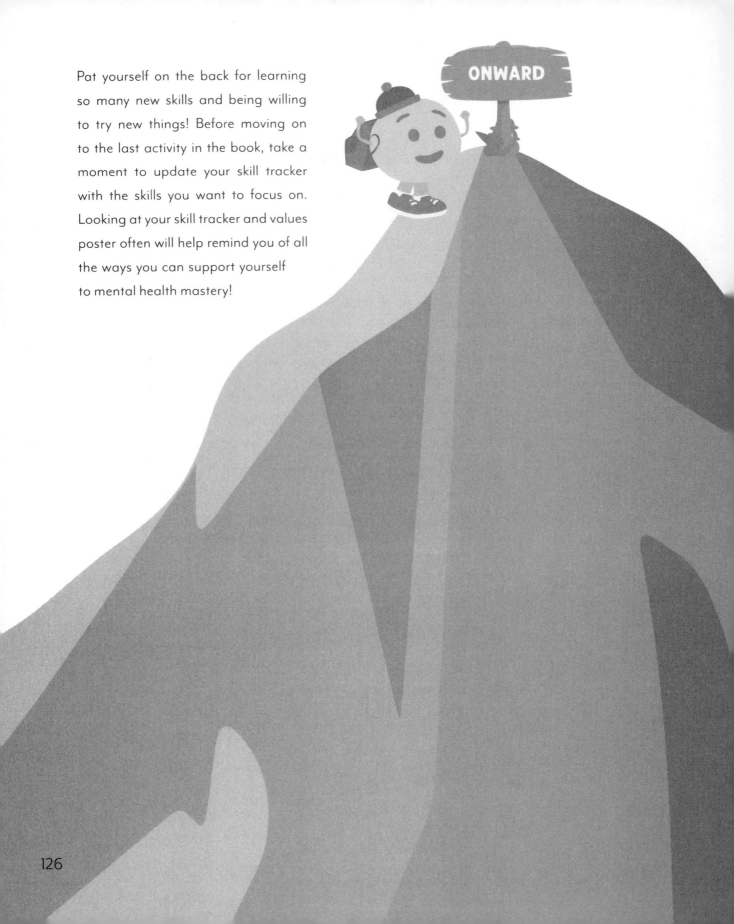

Pat yourself on the back for learning so many new skills and being willing to try new things! Before moving on to the last activity in the book, take a moment to update your skill tracker with the skills you want to focus on. Looking at your skill tracker and values poster often will help remind you of all the ways you can support yourself to mental health mastery!

ONWARD

LETTER FROM THE TOP

Well, adventurer, you're now ready to leave Preteen Peak and continue with your journey up to the summit.

Take a few minutes to look at your vision board. Close your eyes and imagine you're living the adult life you dream of. You've overcome every obstacle in your path and are thriving using the skills you've learned to master your mental health. Write yourself a letter from the top of the mountain, encouraging yourself to keep going when things are difficult, or the path forward is uncertain.

Dear preteen me,

_____

_____

_____

_____

_____

_____

_____

_____

_____

_____

_____

_____

_____

You've got this; keep going.

With admiration,
Future you

ADDITIONAL RESOURCES

SKILL TRACKER

Learn to master your mental health one skill at a time!

Write each skill below and color a box each day you practice it.

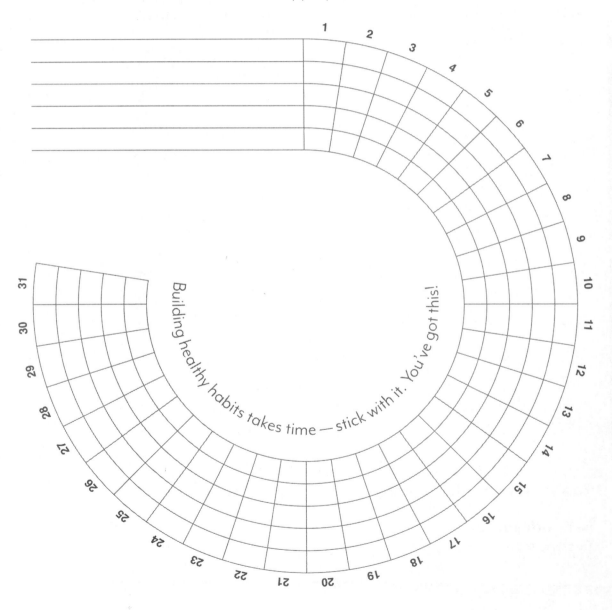

Building healthy habits takes time — stick with it. You've got this!

SKILL LIST

Here's a list of all the skills you've learned throughout this book. Use it to remind you of everything you can do to overcome challenges and keep your mental health on track. Check the skills you have and the skills or information you need to solve your problem. Then make a plan, or ask for help to build the skills and get the information you need. Keep practicing new skills daily until they feel easier and more automatic.

- Add to your **vision board** to inspire you to keep going.

- Use your **strengths** to help you solve problems.

- Practice building your **hopefulness** that things can and will change.

- Practice building your **willingness** to try new things.

- Practice building your **confidence** in your ability to cope.

- Practice coming off autopilot: **Notice what's going on** in the thinking, feeling, and doing parts of your brain.

- Notice when you're using a **short-term avoidance strategy**, come up with an alternative coping strategy, and practice using it.

- When difficult feelings come up, **notice them and practice accepting them** (name it to tame it, feel it to heal it).

- Get your **sleep schedule** on track.

- Nourish your brain and body with **good food**.

- **Use movement/exercise** to help your body feel its best and reduce stress.

- Revisit your **wellness plan** and increase your self-care.

- Use mindfulness to **notice and be curious** about what is happening here and now.

- Separate yourself from **unhelpful or unkind thoughts**.

- **Treat yourself** the way you would treat a good friend.

- **Write a compassionate letter** to yourself.

- Look at your **mindful moments journal** to remind yourself of the good things in life.

- **Hunt for positive things** to add to your "highlight of my day" jar or gratitude journal.

- **Use your flexible brain** to find creative solutions to your problem.

- **Add the word "YET"** to your fixed thoughts ("I can't...", "I'll never...") to remind you that things can change.

- Check **the balance of your thoughts**—what's the ratio of positive, neutral, and negative thoughts?

- Take off your doom and gloom glasses so you can **focus on the positive and neutral things** in your life.

- Identify any **thinking ruts** you may be falling into—and be kind to yourself when you do.

- Use the **"is it true?"/"is it helpful?"/"is it kind?"** filter to get your thoughts back on track.

- Remember that **thoughts are not facts** (and you're not a duck!).

- Pause and **choose to move toward the life you want** and what's important to you.

- **Do a body scan** to notice what emotions are visiting you, and how they feel in your body.

- **Get curious** about what messages your emotions have for you.

- **Use the pain x resistance = suffering equation** to notice and reduce your resistance.

- **Use self-compassion** to accept the painful things in life and make yourself as comfortable as you can be while the pain is present.

- **Make and use a care package** to comfort yourself.

- **Remind yourself of all the special people** who have been part of your journey so far.

- **Reach out to a close friend** for connection and support.

- Check if **your boundaries** are being tested or crossed.

- Assertively **communicate your boundaries** and needs.

- Remember that relationships are going to change—which is hard but okay. **Use self-compassion** when you're feeling grief or loss.

- **Let your parents/caregivers** or other trusted adults **know** what's going on with you—they are there to help you.

- Work on your relationship with yourself—**be your own best friend**.

- **Clarify your values**—what matters most to you right now?

- **Use your values** to help you make decisions.

- **Behave according to your values**.

- **Break goals into small steps** to help you get started.

- Remember that failure means you've succeeded at trying. **Be willing to fail** often.

- Review the main influences in your life—**keep the helpful, ditch the harmful**.

- Ask someone who is **a helpful and trusted influence** for guidance and advice.

- Write down the parts of the problem that are in your control and the parts that are not in your control. **Focus on controlling what you can and accepting the rest.**

- Is the problem as big as you think? Put things in perspective and **pick the skill that will support you the best.**

EMOTIONAL WEATHER CHART

Color a box each day to see how your feelings change over time.

MONTH:						
1						
2						
3						
4						
5						
6						
7						
8						
9						
10						
12						
13						
14						
15						

HOW DO YOU FEEL TODAY?

☀	joyful / happy / silly / content / great
🌧	sad / lonely / insecure / depressed / numb
🌬	productive / energetic / motivated / active
⛅	average / normal / chill / good
⛈	angry / anxious / frustrated / annoyed
🌫	tired / lazy / bored / dull

16						
17						
18						
19						
20						
21						
22						
23						
24						
25						
26						
27						
28						
29						
30						
31						

HOW DO YOU FEEL TODAY?

	joyful happy silly content great
	sad lonely insecure depressed numb
	productive energetic motivated active
	average normal chill good
	angry anxious frustrated annoyed
	tired lazy bored dull

133

HELP REQUEST CARD

Dear Trusted Adult,

If a young person has given you this page, they need help with a serious issue that's tricky to talk about. Please take time to read what they have written below and support them to get help from their family doctor or youth mental health service.

* * *

Name: Date:

I need help with:

- Food/eating/body image concerns

- Self-harm

- Suicidal thoughts

- Bullying/cyberbullying

- Safety/care at home

- Other: _____

This has been a serious problem for me for (please circle):

Less than 1 month   1 to 3 months   3 to 6 months   6 to 12 months   More than 1 year

I have/have not spoken to anyone about this before. (circle one)

* * *

Thanks for being a safe and trusted adult in this young person's life and for taking their mental health seriously.

REFERENCES

Beck, J. S. (2020). *Cognitive Behavior Therapy: Basics and Beyond, Third Edition.* The Guilford Press.

Harris, R. (2022). *The Happiness Trap: How to Stop Struggling and Start Living, Second Edition.* Shambhala.

Neff, K. (2011). *Self-Compassion: The Proven Power of Being Kind to Yourself.* William Morrow.

Siegel, D. J., & Bryson, T. P. (2011). *The Whole-Brain Child.* Delacorte Press.

Lisa Shetler, MPsych, is a child, adolescent, and family clinical psychologist based in Australia with over a decade of experience spent supporting the mental health of middle schoolers as they face the specific challenges of this developmental period. She works directly with young people, their families, and schools in her large group practice—Flow Psychology and Therapeutic Services—where she also provides training, supervision, assessment, and group programs. Flow's website and social media have a wide reach to both local and international audiences seeking information relating to child psychology. Find out more at www.flowpsych.com.au.

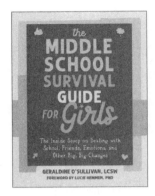
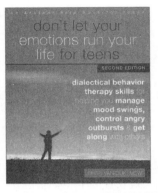
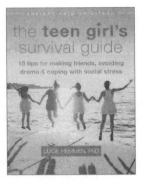
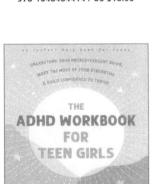
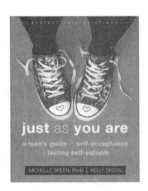
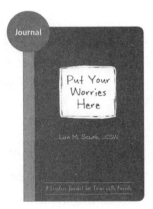
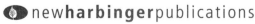